THE MAGICAL AND RITUAL USE OF
PERFUMES

THE MAGICAL AND RITUAL USE OF
PERFUMES

Richard Alan Miller and Iona Miller

Illustrated by Toni L. Taylor

DESTINY BOOKS

Rochester, Vermont

Destiny Books
One Park Street
Rochester, Vermont 05767
www.DestinyBooks.com

Copyright © 1990 by Richard Miller and Iona Miller

All rights reserved. No part of this book may be reproduced or utilized in any form or by any means, electronic or mechanical, including photocopying, recording, or by any information storage and retrieval system, without permission in writing from the publisher.

LIBRARY OF CONGRESS CATALOGING-IN-PUBLICATION DATA

Miller, Richard.
    The magical and ritual use of perfumes.

    Bibliography: p.
    Includes index.
    1. Perfumes—Miscellanea. 2. Occultism. 3. Cabala.
I. Miller, Iona.   II. Title.
BF1442.P47M54   1988   133   88-32020

ISBN: 978-0-89281-210-3

Printed and bound in the United States

13

Destiny Books is a division of Inner Traditions International

Grateful acknowledgment to the publishers listed below for permission to reprint excerpts from the following:

The Homeric Hymns, tr. Charles Boer, second revised edition (Dallas: Spring Publications, Inc., 1979), © 1970 by Charles Boer.
777 and Other Qabalistic Writings of Aleister Crowley, Aleister Crowley (York Beach, ME: Samuel Weiser, 1973), pp. 113–20.
Transcendental Magic, Eliphas Levi (York Beach, ME: Samuel Weiser, 1970), pp. 252–4. Used by permission of the publisher.
Transcendental Magic, Eliphas Levi (London: Century Hutchinson Limited).

Dedicated with love to our daughter, Charissa

*It is only with scent and silk and artifices
that we raise love from an instinct to a passion.*

—George Moore

ACKNOWLEDGMENTS

Special thanks are due to magical perfumer Lady Sara Cunningham-Carter for her illuminating conversation and years of qabalistic experimentation.

Thanks to Lotte Lieb of Stellar Visions for sharing her formulae and their derivations.

Thanks also to Kirk Bergman of Nu Essence, a special friend and alchemist.

TABLE OF CONTENTS

PREFACE		xi
INTRODUCTION		1
Chapter 1	PERFUME MAGIC: THE ESSENCE OF REALITY	3
Chapter 2	ESSENCE AND QUINTESSENCE: PERFUMERY AND ALCHEMY	11
Chapter 3	INTRODUCTION TO THE MATERIALS OF PERFUMERY	15
Chapter 4	THE LANGUAGE OF PERFUME	22
Chapter 5	THE ESSENCE OF THE QABALA	31
	1. KETHER = AMBERGRIS	37
	2. CHOKMAH = MUSK	41
	3. BINAH = MYRRH, CIVET	45
	4. CHESED = CEDAR	51
	5. GEBURAH = TOBACCO, LEATHER	55
	6. TIPHARETH = OLIBANUM	59
	7. NETZACH = BENZOIN, ROSE, SANDALWOOD	63
	8. HOD = STORAX	69
	9. YESOD = JASMINE	73
	10. MALKUTH = PATCHOULI, DITTANY OF CRETE	77
Chapter 6	THE ESSENCE OF THE PATHS	79
	KEY 11 = THE FOOL = GALBANUM	81
	KEY 12 = THE MAGICIAN = MASTIC, STORAX	83
	KEY 13 = THE HIGH PRIESTESS = CAMPHOR, ALOE	85
	KEY 14 = THE EMPRESS = SANDALWOOD, MYRTLE	87
	KEY 15 = THE EMPEROR = BASIL	89
	KEY 16 = THE HIEROPHANT = STORAX, VANILLA	91
	KEY 17 = THE LOVERS = WORMWOOD	92
	KEY 18 = THE CHARIOT = ONYCHA (LABDANUM)	94
	KEY 19 = STRENGTH/LUST = OLIBANUM	96
	KEY 20 = THE HERMIT = NARCISSUS	97
	KEY 21 = THE WHEEL OF FORTUNE = SAFFRON	99
	KEY 22 = ADJUSTMENT = GALBANUM, MINT	101
	KEY 23 = THE HANGED MAN = ONYCHA, MYRRH	103
	KEY 24 = DEATH = BENZOIN, OPOPONAX	104
	KEY 25 = TEMPERANCE/ART = ALOE	106
	KEY 26 = THE DEVIL = MUSK, CIVET, (BAY)	107
	KEY 27 = THE TOWER = PEPPER	108
	KEY 28 = THE STAR = GALBANUM, BERGAMOT	109
	KEY 29 = THE MOON = AMBERGRIS, VIOLET	111
	KEY 30 = THE SUN = OLIBANUM, CINNAMON	112
	KEY 31 = JUDGEMENT/THE AEON = OLIBANUM	114
	KEY 32 = THE UNIVERSE = CYPRESS	115

Chapter 7   PLANETARY PERFUMES AND THEIR
            GOD-FORMS   117
    THE SUN = APOLLO   125
    THE MOON = ARTEMIS   129
    MERCURY = HERMES   133
    VENUS = APHRODITE   137
    MARS = ARES   141
    JUPITER = ZEUS   145
    SATURN = HERA   149
    URANUS = URANUS   151
    NEPTUNE = POSEIDON   155
    PLUTO = HADES   157

SUPPLIERS   158

BIBLIOGRAPHY   164

APPENDIX   166

INGREDIENT INDEX   167

INDEX   169

PREFACE

The philosophical basis of this book originates in the Western occult tradition. Magic and ritual are one answer to the modern search for meaningful experience. The goal of the Western occult tradition has been to understand the arts and sciences. In the not so distant past, such comprehensive education was understood to have definite metaphysical implications: it meant not only knowledge of the nature of things but of oneself. Concerned with stimulating latent abilities and creating new resources for themselves, occult practitioners have continued throughout time to learn systematically about the worlds without and within themselves.

Perhaps the most systematic method of self-understanding developed originally in the Hebrew culture. The system, known as the Qabala, provided clear guidelines for self-development and enhanced spirituality. The practice of qabalistic theory is based on the circuit of the Tree of Life, which provides a map of the inner realms (see Figure 1). Its ten spheres and thirty-two paths are "stations" on the inner journey. The Qabala is not only a Jewish heritage. Commerce led to exchange of beliefs among ancient peoples. Qabalistic thought eventually fused with Egyptian, Gnostic, Christian, and Oriental elements, making it a very broad-based world-view.

Because so much of ancient science was not empirical but metaphysical, the practices of astrology, alchemy, and magic corresponded to the processes represented on the Tree of Life. The evolution of this eclectic system culminated in the eighteenth and nineteenth centuries with the formation of such groups as the Rosicrucians, Masons, and less well-known occult groups, such as the Order of the Golden Dawn. These groups synthesized the disparate elements of the Western mystical tradition into a coherent whole.

Magicians such as Paracelsus, John Dee, Eliphas Levi, S.L. McGregor Mathers, Dion Fortune, A.E. Waite, and Aleister Crowley brought these ancient traditions into print. In many works, the magical and ritual use of perfumes was a key element. The magical connections of perfumes to states of consciousness were distilled from ancient Egyptians; Arabian alchemists; Greek, Hindu, and Buddhist ceremony; and the lore of various cultures.

What did these magicians feel they got from this art? The use of such symbols as perfumes gave them

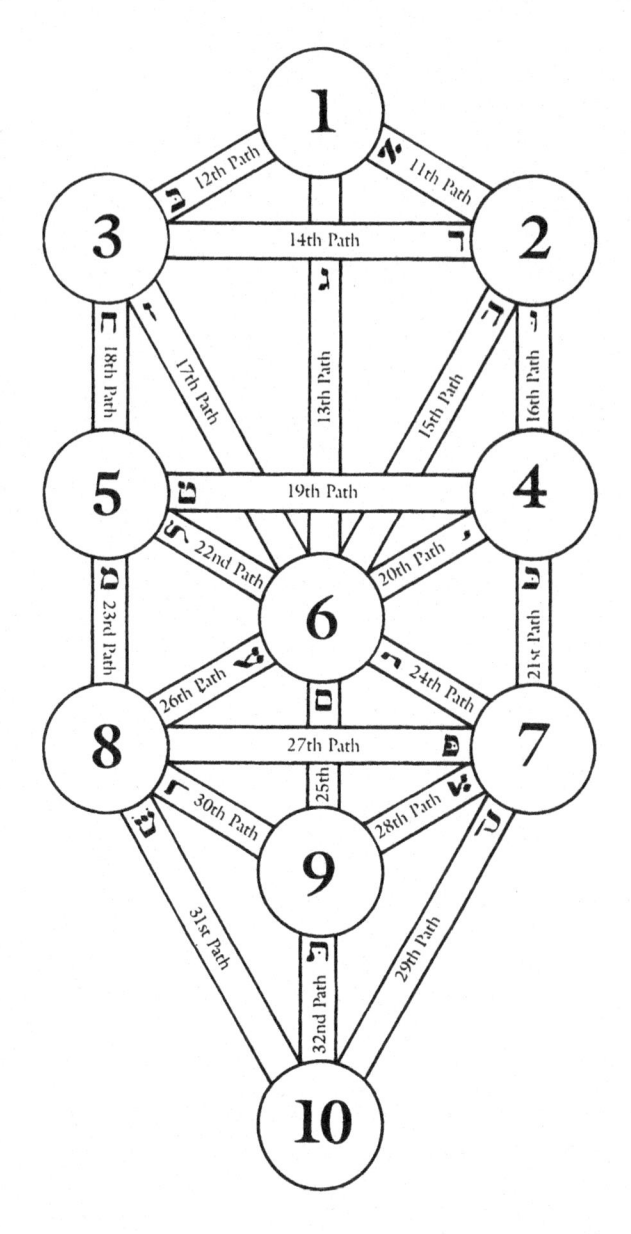

Figure 1. The Tree of Life
The aspirant climbs the tree beginning from Sphere 10, the most material level, up to Sphere 1, reunion with godhead. The other spheres represent the intervening mystical states.

a key to unlock the subconscious, providing a means of integrating new qualities and improving their lives. Without knowing the specifics of modern neuroanatomy they realized that scents had the power to evoke an experience of the astral plane when properly employed.

Qabala provides a paradigm or thought model for the aspirant. The holistic nature of the Qabala is realized through the system of correspondences, which includes not only perfumes, but a wider range of symbols.* For example, the sphere *Tiphareth* on the Tree of Life, which symbolizes union with the Holy Guardian Angel, includes much more than the fragrance frankincense. It is also the sun in astrology; gold in alchemy; the godforms Christ, Mithras, and Ra; the colors yellow and gold; the animals phoenix and lion; the stones topaz and yellow diamond; and so forth. Combined in ritual or in imagination, these diverse symbols create the desired atmosphere or state of consciousness.

The synthesis that draws from both Western and Eastern esoteric systems is known as the Hermetic Qabala. A stepchild of Jewish mysticism, it is relevant to those of all nations and belief systems. The qabalistic techniques of self-development were clarified in the Renaissance with a major shift in emphasis from will power to imagination. Scent is a powerful stimulus for the imagination: it evokes visual images, sounds, memories, and emotions. The magical use of scent exploits this natural process systematically, creating positive change.

Much as people develop a keen aesthetic appreciation for gourmet food or fine wines, we can acquire a deeper understanding of the role of our olfactory sense. This is a small but important step in our quest for wholeness. The magical and ritual use of perfumes is so fundamental in both primitive and sophisticated societies that it may be a basic drive in man. It is a crosscultural phenomenon the traditions of which have been given little attention in our busy society. An introduction to the magical uses of fragrance can be very enriching.

Modern research in neuroanatomy shows that scents provide direct access to the emotional part of the brain and memory. Scents evoke visual images, and visual images are always accompanied by somatic patterns—a set of bodily feelings and tensions with cognitive or experiential meaning. Smells, especially those encountered repeatedly, are stored in the memory as holistic scent impressions. When an odor is smelled again, even years later, it can call forth a host of associations, as Arthur Symons reveals in "Memory":

> As a perfume doth remain
> In the folds where it has lain
> So the thought of you, remaining
> Deeply folded in my brain,
> Will not leave me, all things leave me
> You remain. . . .

The associations a scent calls up can link the body and mind in a unique manner. Modern theories of imagery confirm the ancient notions of healing and transformation: the sensory components of an image include the tactile, gustatory, visual, auditory, and olfactory. The olfactory aspect of the image gives the quickest recall of an emotional response and its meaning. Manipulating the entire image once it is called up can produce creative change in the body and the emotions.

---

*Note: The Qabala is a vast field of experimentation in which many authors disagree within a generally accepted framework. The authors have done their best to offer correspondences based on both tradition and personal experimentation.

INTRODUCTION

From time immemorial incense, perfume, and sweet-smelling herbs have played an important part in religion and magic. Their legendary virtues fill many books. Exotic scents have charmed and lured men and women, but this is not the aspect of fragrance dealt with here. Rather, the alchemy of scent deals mainly with the ability of aromas to evoke psychological and sensory responses.

This inner mystery of the sacred science of scent discloses perfumes as the royal road to the subconscious. Truly magical perfume formulae work on both the conscious and subconscious mind to elicit a specific predetermined response. This book will help you understand and experience which scents call forth which responses.

Certain scents are so uplifting that their divine essence seems to carry us to transcendent realms. These heavenly scents waft us out of ordinary existence to a momentary state of rapture. Since this state is above or removed from ordinary consciousness, it is called superconsciousness. Magicians speak of this exalted state of mind in reference to the Higher Self or Inner Guide. Psychologists call it an experience of the archetype of the Self. This self-realization is a temporary feeling of oneness or rightness with the universe.

Specific formulae not only call forth predictable responses, they can also condition our consciousness through association. Research shows that we all respond consciously and unconsciously to the stimuli of sound, color, and scent. Certain scents cause us to react emotionally or physically. Some scents stimulate the sexual centers, others are soothing to the nerves; some activate the psychic centers, still others have healing properties.

Used properly, these scents can stimulate our physical, emotional, mental, and spiritual selves in a seemingly magical way. This book is designed to provide a hands-on working knowledge of formulae and blending procedures. You will learn when and how to utilize your fragrance creations. With these tools you can experiment with this ancient art form, enhancing your olfactory awareness and your spiritual growth. Perfumery is an alchemical art that allows the imagination free play, much as the performing and graphic arts do. Used in conjunction with ritual in a self-directed program of psychological growth, it is a potent tool.

Using this book for a guide, you will gain the ability to begin immediately combining original fragrances for various uses. Needless to say, creating your own unique blends can be a joy for yourself and for those to whom you give or sell them. Besides employing traditional recipes, you can create unique fragrances for individuals based on their astrological charts. These can be used as *signature* perfumes, describing the quintessence of the individual. Alternatively, your blends can include ingredients designed to balance the personality by stimulating qualities that are absent.

You may wonder where the basic ingredients come from. The array of products offered in today's market as raw materials vary greatly in terms of source and quality. How can any beginner in this field hope to know which oils are quality products, much less those that are "magical"?

A good rule of thumb is to buy from reputable suppliers and to buy the finest products you can afford. In perfumery the quality of the pure essential oil determines the quality of the blend. Pure, natural oils are the best, and the presence of any solvents or adulterants should be clearly noted. Some perfume oil suppliers cut their oils by one-third with an oil solvent and the quality may be poor to start with. If you use a middleman to get a decent price or a smaller quantity of oil, make sure that company purchases from a reliable source. Good quality is important to the retailer, hobbyist, and practicing mystic, though for widely varying reasons. Some of the top houses are Berje, Belmay, Norda (Division of PPF International), and Givaudan. (See the appendix for a complete listing).

Select a good supplier or you will be disappointed with the results. There are many cheap essential oils available for potpourri and room freshening. Any magic they contain is in their names rather than in the products. However, if a person truly believes an oil is magical, then that belief will, in fact, impart some charge to the essence. One obvious solution is to add a knowledge of the correspondences and planetary rulerships of the various herbs, spices, and essential oils. By making your own compounds you are assured of good products, and you will know what is in them.

In ancient times all religious or magical incenses—quite unlike today's powdered varieties—

were made from natural herbs, spices, and resins. Each of these substances was considered to share a common essence with a certain planetary power. Bay, cinnamon, frankincense, and marigold, for example, are all attributed to the sun, and they mediate its quality to us. In other words, these scents create a psychological reaction in us that can be seen as awakening latent solar potentials.

Tapping this potential, we can use scents as a language for communicating with our sub- and superconscious energies. To carry on the analogy, solar scents can be used to evoke an emotional experience of the higher Self, symbol of integration. We think that is the reason the Catholic church employs frankincense in its rituals. Christ is a solar hero in the language of symbolism. Solar scents can also be used to stimulate creativity.

It has been said that there are no amateur perfumers, but we should not be daunted in our exploration of this realm. The main qualities the aspiring perfumer needs are sustained enthusiasm and plain old hard work. Even an amateur perfumer can make attractive blends, but for more sophisticated fragrances one needs experience. You can learn to acquire a larger scent memory by routinely smelling, thinking, compounding, testing, rejecting, reconsidering. This is the process of composing an olfactory symphony. No amount of reading or theory can substitute for the experience gained through practice.

Perfumery has been the most neglected of the Hermetic arts. This may be because olfaction accounts for only about 2% of our sensory input, and 98% of that small amount is subliminal. Most of our sensory information comes in through our eyes, and we are quite conscious of it. The subliminal stimulation we derive from scents, however, is potent because it reaches right into our subconscious: it affects our emotional nature.

The bridge of the nose is the only place where the brain is directly exposed to the environment. Early cultures recognized the mysterious effects exerted over them by fragrant substances. They extended their delight at these scents and supposed that their gods likewise enjoyed them. They deduced that heaven surely must be filled with luxurious olfactory delights.

Chapter 1

PERFUME MAGIC: THE ESSENCE OF REALITY

Perfumes and incenses have always been employed in magical rites, and the ancient Thaumaturgists made an especial study of the physical and moral reaction of different odors.

—Israel Regardie, *The Tree of Life*

Essence—the primal element. The word has long been associated with both soul and fragrance. The essence of any substance reveals its fundamental, characteristic nature. The magical essence of a human being, in psychological terms, is the higher self. Magic is the quest for union with this inner divinity by the use of the imagination. Referring to this higher Self, magician Aleister Crowley informs us, "Every man and every woman is a Star." In his 1892 compendium, *Lexicon alchemiae*, Martin Ruland identifies Self and imagination when he states, "Imagination is the star in man, the celestial or supercelestial body."

In *Psychology and Alchemy* C. G. Jung points out that the imagination is related to essence.

> The singular expression "astrum" (star) is a Paracelsan term, which in this context means something like "quintessence." Imagination is therefore a concentrated extract of the life forces, both physical and psychic. . . . he [the aspirant] works with and through his own quintessence and is himself the indispensable condition of his own experiment.

The practice of natural magic involves experimentation with the imaginal faculty. According to Jung, Paracelsus equated the "spirit of the fifth essence" with the "spirit of truth" and the "clarified body." At the same time he reveals that he draws from the wisdom of the Qabala and recommends the practice to his students:

> . . . bear in mind if you wish to apply all these things, that you take to yourselves the religion of the Cabal and walk in its light, for the Cabal is well-founded. Ask and it will be granted to you, knock, you will be heard and it will be opened unto you. From this granting and opening there will flow what you desire: you will see into the lowest depths of the earth, into the depths of hell, into the third heaven.

You will gain more wisdom than Solomon, you will have greater communion with God than Moses and Aaron.

Magic is the practice of practical qabalism. It involves the process of changing yourself through imagination. Its goal is the same as that of psychological therapy, but it does not stop with mental well-being. Magic is a process of using the creative imagination to achieve a high level of spiritual well-being.

The essence of magic lies in psychosensory evocation or stimulation of the mind and body in a highly specific manner. The magician's use of ritual and an elaborate correspondence system is actually a form of communication with higher levels of being. Through this medium he communes with his subconscious mind (Jung's "depths of the earth"), his higher self ("the third heaven"), and possibly with entities from other dimensions of the imaginal realm.

Since ancient times, the same god has been said to preside over both communication and the practice of magic. In Egypt this god was called Thoth, in Greece Hermes, in Rome Mercury. Scent is one form of communication. We are reminded that there is not only a language of perfumes, but that there is emotional magic in perfumes and in smells in general. Odors can change our moods, bring memories back to consciousness, arouse sexual desire, and generally make life more pleasant.

Odors are potent in their influence because they operate on us at a subconscious or subliminal level. Thus, their influence on our emotional nature bypasses the critical mind. Unlike our other senses, smell is a chemical sense, requiring the transfer of odoriferous molecules as the primary source of information. Smell impulses take the fastest, most direct route to the brain, even quicker than visual or auditory processing. Furthermore, these impulses travel directly to the brain's limbic system, which governs emotion. Using perfumes as fumigations in ritual therefore provides us with direct access to preprogrammed emotional states.

We can use scents as access codes to specific altered states of consciousness by employing them as olfactory "anchors." *Anchoring* refers to the tendency for any one element of an experience—including visual, auditory, kinesthetic, olfactory and gustatory components—to bring back the entire experience. Since a scent memory is actually retained longer (and undergoes less distortion) than a visual memory, smells are particularly effective anchors. Each time we repeat the use of a particular scent in a ritual setting, we can enter that particular frame of mind more quickly and more deeply. Soon, the scent alone evokes the amalgamation of memories of all the rituals done under its influence.

One modern science of communication, neurolinguistic programming (NLP), is frequently equated with magic in popular literature. NLP recognizes three main styles of perception: visual, auditory, and kinesthetic (feeling). It also classifies some rare persons as using olfactory information as their primary mode of perception. These people literally sniff out information about their environment. An example is the innovative therapist and founder of conjoint family therapy, Virginia Satir. She actually uses her nose to monitor the emotional state of clients in therapy!

Anyone can train this much neglected sense: the sense of smell grows sharper with practice. If we educate our noses and overcome our programming to ignore this stimulation, we can tap our full smell potential. Scientists have found that our skill at identifying odors peaks between the ages of 20 to 40, tapers off from ages 40 to 70, then declines rapidly. The average person can name about 70% of all odors, but most of us have odor blind spots, or areas where we cannot pinpoint odors easily accessible to others. One reason we are imprecise in describing or identifying odors is that we lack an extensive vocabulary for odors, but with practice we can learn to detect subtleties.

Perfumes are important in the ritual setting because odors are automatically coded in memory as whole images. When you remember a smell it also brings back how things looked, sounded, felt, and even tasted. Thus scents function as the "essence of reality"—an even more powerful emotional trigger than music.

This little-known secret technique will be even more important in the near future for self-conducted therapy, or the simple process of changing ourselves. Right now, fragrance and flavor chemists are working on perfumes to help ease stress. Because smell is a chemical sense we will eventually be able to design odors to produce specific effects.

Perhaps these evocative fragrances are already here, as the magical perfumes. Properly employed, they are keys to altered states of consciousness. Any sensory stimulus that triggers an internal response can be an anchor; but scents are especially useful because of their manner of encoding experience holistically. Just remember the salt-spray smell of the ocean, or the smell of the damp, balsamic forest, and you are there in your imagination.

Neuroanatomists tell us that, unlike the other senses, the olfactory cells send their data to that part of the brain thought to be the oldest in evolutionary terms. This system—the limbic system—deals with the regulation of motor activities and primitive drives. Stimulation of the olfactory bulb sends signals to the amygdala, the area of the brain concerned with visceral and behavioral mechanisms, especially those associated with sensory and sexual functions. Smells directly influence the digestive system, sexual arousal, and emotional behavior.

Families can actually identify one another by scent alone, research shows. Siblings can detect one another with remarkable accuracy. Mothers can recognize their offspring. Nursing infants can distinguish their mother's milk from others. Apparently we each have an "odor signature" created by our body fats and other chemicals.

Research shows that women can discriminate odors more acutely than men. When their estrogen levels rise, their noses are even more sensitive. The sense of smell of both men and women is duller in the morning and keener at night. Scientist attribute women's special abilities in part to better verbal skills: if we can correctly label and encode a smell, the chances of identifying it later are better.

We can become familiar with the language of scent. From ancient times, certain scents have been reserved for certain gods. A granite tablet on the breast of the great Sphinx of Egypt depicts King Thothmes IV offering incense and scented oil to the gods. In modern psychology, these gods are termed *archetypes*, and each has its unique qualities. Human aspects of these archetypes include psychological qualities, feelings, and behavior patterns (mental, emotional, and psychic levels). Therefore, if specific scents are associated with these archetypes, we should be able to invoke them, or call them up, by the use of perfumes in ritual. This calling forth of the god was one reason for using incense and perfumes in ritual.

RITUAL ENACTMENT

In ritual, you are trying to align yourself with some higher quality or resource you seek to infuse into your personality. At least, this is one use of ritual. In formulating and performing the rite you include visual, auditory, olfactory (perfume/incense) and gustatory (the eucharist) elements. Since it is the nature of a scent to encode the gestalt of an experience, after you have performed a rite enough to make a clear memory of it, merely smelling the associated scent should anchor that quality into your daily life. You can employ the Qabala systematically in this way, to arouse inner resources, using scent to magically fortify yourself until the qualities are ingrained.

If you wanted to stimulate your psychic abilities or powers of ESP (extrasensory perception), for example, you could do a standard banishing ritual (see Exercise A, page 6) followed by an invocation of the moon (or Great White Goddess), using her characteristic scents of jasmine, camphor, or aloes, depending on which level you wanted to invoke—the psychic-sexual center or the Blessed Virgin aspect, the third eye. During the height of the ritual, you identify yourself consciously with the qualities you are seeking, aligning your personality with this aspect of the higher self. Conclude the ritual with a Middle Pillar exercise (see Exercise B, page 8) and banishing rite.

Once you have performed enough rituals to be able to imagine yourself doing them in your mind's eye, you are a minor adept. At this point you can put yourself in the altered state of consciousness at will and operate exclusively on the astral plane, so to speak. When you can do this, the use of the perfume alone as the sole physical stimulus to get into the mood will be very effective. You will no longer need to tote around a plethora of magical appurtenances to contact your superconscious. Anchoring allows you to build bridges between contexts and resources.

Exercise A CIRCLE MAGIC AND BANISHING RITUAL

Building the circle or sphere of light around oneself is the simplest form of magical ritual. It is an affirmation of one's wholeness and active participation in the cosmos. The circle is a universal symbol of the feminine, while the penetrating shaft of light has a masculine quality.

Ritual is an end itself. It is a celebration of life; it is the soul in action. During ritual we alter our consciousness in accordance with the symbols being used. The magical circle, or mandala, with its four quarters relates us to our environment with a maximum of meaning. It gives us physical and spiritual orientation.

The power perimeter is formed by first tracing the circle around oneself, either physically or vividly in the imagination. Next, perform the Qabalistic Cross by picturing a brilliant, piercing ray of scintillating light entering from above your head and grounding through your feet. Then cross yourself from left to right with a horizontal beam of light. Finish with a moment of contemplation with arms crossed over the breast.

Continue with the Banishing Ritual, which will further focus or concentrate your attention within your sacred precinct. Facing east, stretch out your dominant hand, either holding your magical sword (or dagger) or pointing your index finger. This can be performed "on the astral" via visualization if you can hold the picture clearly.

Trace a pentagram with your outstretched hand; watch it burst into flame. Then fling it forth into the east until it disappears in the far distance. Intone the god-name YHVH (yod-heh-vav-heh). Turn north, repeat the gestures, and use the name AGLA (ah-ge-lah). Do the same in the west, saying AHIH (eh-he-yeh). Finally, turn south, fling out the pentagram, and intone ADNI (ah-doh-nai).

Return to your position facing east. Extend your arms in the form of a cross, and say, "Before me Raphael." This is the archangel of aspiration, pictured as a vast figure clad in billowing yellow light, scintillating with mauve or violet. Feel a cool wind emanating from this entity, awakening your potential.

Turn south, saying, "To the south Michael." This angel of fire is a muscular warrior clad in robes of brilliant red, scintillating with green. You feel intense radiation emanating from this angel of inspiration.

Facing west, call out, "To the west Gabriel." Archangel of water, he holds out a blue chalice of ambrosial elixir. Sea tides surge around his feet and you smell the moisture of the spray. Gabriel is a purifying energy.

Finally, turn north, intoning, "To the north Auriel," and feel the stabilizing energy of this broad-shouldered, placid figure. He is clad in indigo with glittering flashes of gold. Picture him in verdant fields of grain and flowers. The golden orb and sickle in his outstretched arms symbolize peace.

To close your operation, repeat the Qabalistic Cross. Remember to open any ritual with this cleansing and focusing, but also use it to close a circle and dissipate the concentration of energy and return yourself to normal awareness. This ceremonial awakening back into everyday life makes an important distinction between sacred and profane experience.

Learn more about this ritual in Israel Regardie's *The Middle Pillar*.

Ritual magic, done with the proper attitude, is actually a form of self-hypnosis. The great benefit of hypnosis in general over casual memory or regular talk therapies is that it allows you full emotional participation, bypassing the critical mind. This permits a true catharsis. It is a very potent tool for changing yourself in a prearranged direction. You can use it for acquiring formerly unavailable resources that can be quite useful in your daily life. And, as we have shown, scents in particular open up direct access to the emotional part of the brain, which has the greatest impact on the autonomic nervous system and the subconscious mind.

In fact, if you have a vivid imagination, you need never act out a ritual on the physical plane. By simply taking a few deep breaths and establishing a regular pattern of rhythmic breathing, then visualizing yourself going through the banishing ritual, you perform an excellent induction for self-hypnosis. Some prefer to call this technique *guided imagery*. One of the main symbols of the Egyptian god Thoth was the all-seeing single eye, the mind's eye of imagination.

During your trance experience, always keep the perspective of operating within your astral body—your self as seen or experienced in the imagination. Do not just be a spectator. You need to be feeling the sensation of movement and experiencing with your senses as if it were all quite physical. The only exception to these guidelines occurs when you want to distance yourself from something you are finding intolerably unpleasant. Then you mentally move your perspective to viewing the scene as if it were a movie. In normal ritual conditions, you need to feel the heft and weight of your magical sword as you draw the pentagrams. When you draw the perimeter of your magical circle, see it as an impenetrable barrier, impervious to all the external forces of the cosmos. As you visualize the archangels in the various quarters, feel the wind from the east, the heat from the south, the moisture from the west, and the earthy groundedness of the north. Experience the visceral feeling of awe and wonderment all these things inspire in you.

When you drink the wine, feel the cool moisture in your mouth and taste the myriad aromas within the goblet. If you consume a wafer, visualize its charging with light, and as you taste its fullness imagine that light penetrating every aspect of your being. See it . . . hear it . . . feel it . . . taste it . . . smell it . . . then BE IT. Be one with your higher self in that moment of perfection. Then as you circulate that light throughout your entire being during the Middle Pillar exercise, know that you are the light.

COLLAPSING NEGATIVE ANCHORS

Magic is actually the ancient form of psychotherapy, or healing and integration of the mind/body system. We can draw from modern therapy and also from the ancient ritualistic traditions to make a very potent method of healing. Anchors are associations, and we have formed many anchors throughout our lives at random, both positive and negative. Negative associations are known as complexes. These can be used constructively in a ritual setting, if we know how.

In a basic magical ceremony, a circle or sacred precinct is constructed, supposedly to protect one from demonic influence. In Jungian psychology, these demons are translated into modern language as psychological complexes or blocks to further growth. One of these minor demons might be called lack of concentration, or focus. The circle acts like a lens or focus to keep our energy concentrated on one thing and keep out distracting thoughts. Jung identified the magical circle or mandala as a symbol of the self. The banishing ritual clears the psychic atmosphere and then we invoke one pure thought form upon which to concentrate. As stated before, this is actually the induction of self-hypnosis, which is selective awareness.

Hypnosis is not a therapy in itself but rather a tool for getting to the state where work can be done. Once you have cleared a working area the actual magic or process of change begins. You can use techniques from gestalt therapy, NLP, Jungian active imagination, or other therapies in combination with ritual formulae. First, determine on what level you are working: a sexual problem or mother-complex would relate to Yesod (Sphere 9 on the Tree of Life), problems with procrastination to Malkuth (Sphere 10), poor intellectual performance to Hod (Sphere 8), relationship problems to Netzach (Sphere 7), religious dilemmas to Tiphareth (Sphere 6), and so forth.

Now, the work begins in earnest. Go back in time via imagination to an experience where you felt the feeling you want to change. Generally, these are items of unfinished business—things left unsaid, unresolved conflicts, traumas. Relive and intensify that feeling to the point where it is stronger than you have ever felt it before, in real life or memory. Be in that time emotionally, feeling the feeling strongly. See yourself in the experience, hear what went on, feel the body sensations and visceral reactions. Now, anchor all these sensations by gripping your knee in a peculiar way (a way you are not normally touched).

Now invoke the positive qualities of the sphere of the Tree of Life that you wish to incorporate. Remember to invoke only the qualities you want, not the entire effects of the sphere . . . that is too

Exercise B THE MIDDLE PILLAR EXERCISE

Use the Middle Pillar exercise for meditation right after the working period of your ritual. Its primary purpose is to balance out the energies of the mind/body and connect the personality with the higher Self. It establishes a vertical connection between the mundane and the transcendent.

The visualization is based on the primary glyph of the Qabala, which is called the Tree of Life (see graphic at right). By visualizing this figure interpenetrating your body, you align yourself with an image of perfection, both cosmic and terrestrial.

The spheres of the Middle Pillar can be viewed as similar to the eastern concept of chakras. They are visualized as vortices of living light, and each has its symbolic meaning. The top position signifies ineffable divinity, whose energy is drawn into the remainder of the body. The throat-center symbolizes knowledge; the heart-center represents love; the generative-center is the seat of emotions; while the feet represent stability or groundedness.

Each of the centers has one of the five divine names of God attributed to it. No religious or metaphysical theory attaches to the employment of these names. They come from the Judeo-Christian tradition and are offered as audible keys to the different parts of our being. They are an integral part of the rite, which should include visual, aural, and kinesthetic aspects.

Intoning the series of god-names from top to bottom forges a link between the divine genius of the higher Self and the ego or personality. Its goal is to foster self-realization. Doing the Middle Pillar exercise brings in a charge of spiritual force which is realized in your consciousness. Symbolically, it brings godhead into incarnation.

Once you have practiced visualizing the light energy of the various spheres, you may want to add color to your practice. In this case the crown-center is still brilliant white, but the throat-center is pictured as lavender-blue; the heart-center is brilliant gold; the generative-center is violet, while the sphere at the feet is seen as olive green or black.

A full Middle Pillar exercise consists of several phases: the preliminary establishment of rhythmic breathing, the formulation of the five centers through vibrating the god-names, and circulation of the divine force throughout the psychic system.

Circulation of the light distributes the power. Return your attention to the crown. The light then descends the left side of your body and comes up the right side. Then it flows forward over your face, neck, and chest until it reaches the feet and returns to the crown up your back. To wrap up the circulation phase imagine spiraling light surrounding your body. Spiral light up from your feet, wrapping yourself like a mummy. When the light returns to the crown, it shoots out of your head with a brilliant fountain effect.

Regardie calls this exercise the groundwork of all actual developmental work. As the basis of the practice of magic, it creates psychic equilibration of the various human and divine qualities. It is calming, but it also stimulates your potential for creativity. Light permeates the body and produces clarity. Complete your exercise with a banishing ritual to return you to ordinary consciousness.

Learn more about this ritual in Israel Regardie's *The Middle Pillar*.

---

overwhelming. See yourself in the same situation again with all the resources you need to perform and feel the way you want to in the future. Now anchor these positive feelings with another touch.

To neutralize the unpleasant experience forever, all you need do now is to fire off the two anchors simultaneously by recreating both touches in the same moment. This is a highly effective, proven technique, even outside the context of ritual. If you combine a special scent for the sphere, with which you have no other associations, you have a potent mnemonic device for recreating the experience instantaneously. You have changed your associations from unpleasant to pleasant. You have, in effect,

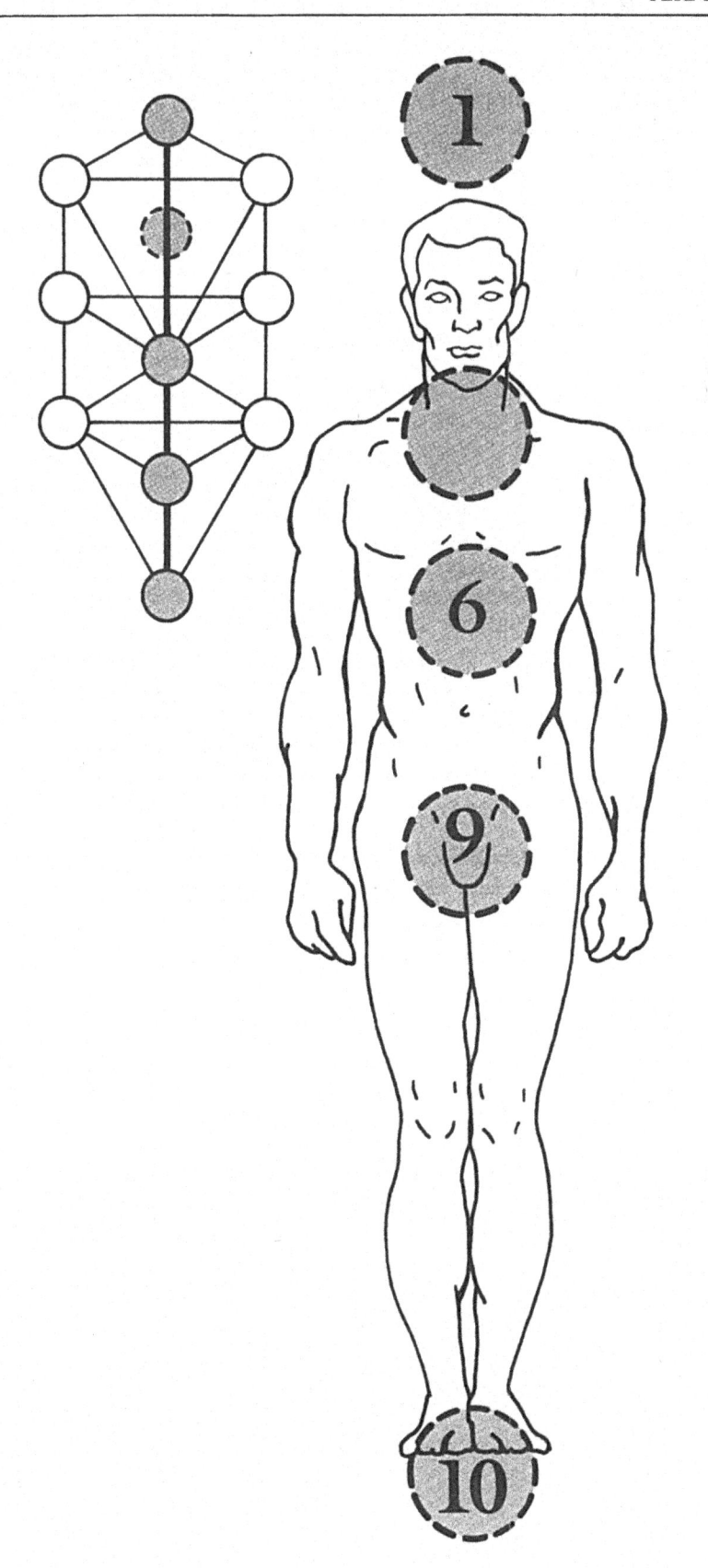

The Middle Pillar

1. Imagine a whirling disk of white light above your head and intone: EH-HE-YEH. Repeat the mantrum ten times.

2. Bring the light down to the throat area where it forms another whirling disk, and intone: YE-HOH-VOH-EL-LOH-HEEM. Repeat three times.

3. Bring the light down to the chest area where it forms another whirling disk and intone: YE-HOH-VOH-EL-OH-AH-VA-DA-AS. Repeat six times.

4. Bring the light down to the genital area and form another whirling disk, and intone: SHA-DAI-EL-CHAI. Repeat nine times.

5. Bring the light down beneath the feet where it forms another whirling disk, and intone: AH-DOH-NAI-HA-AH-RETZ. Repeat ten times.

changed your personal history. Any anchor can be collapsed by another anchor, if the other anchor is of equal or greater intensity, and both are triggered simultaneously.

You can use scents to anchor natural resources and construct resource experiences. You can use your imagination to elicit a sequence of internal states that you have never before experienced. Associate a different touch, or sound, or smell with each step of the sequence. Then fire off the anchors in sequence. Anchor the resulting internal state. Every time you fire off an anchor you get the same response—that is, the quality you've programmed is evoked. This is conditioned response.

SCENT IN RITUAL

Israel Regardie, one of the foremost authors on the Western occult tradition, defines three purposes for the employment of scents in ceremonial magic. The first is "to provide a material vehicle or basis for the manifesting spirit." This requires burning incense to create a dense cloud of smoke upon which the participant imagines the entity. Second, perfumes are offered to the entity being called into communication—most frequently one's Holy Guardian Angel, a symbol of the divine genius or higher Self. In more particularized operations, there are specific scents for each class of being from the inner dimensions, forming calling cards, so to speak.

They are olfactory keys. Finally, there is "the all important intoxicant effect of the powerful and penetrative incenses on the consciousness itself, a separate one being assigned to accompany the invocation of each deity."

Regardie also outlines another means of employing perfumes and incenses by using the Qabala.

Each letter of the Hebrew alphabet has attributed to it a long number of correspondences, of spirits, intelligences, colors, gems, ideas, and incenses. By taking the letters in the name of a spirit, and consulting the proper authorities, a compound of incenses may be made which will spell, through the sense of smell, the name of the spirit. From this compound of perfumes alone the appropriate spirit may be suggested in the imagination and called forth by the proper rites. There can be little doubt as to the essential suggestiveness of these perfumes, since even for ordinary individuals some incenses are definitely seductive and excitant, such as musk and patchouli; yet others overwhelmingly fragrant and generous, and others which are sedative and tranquillizing.

Detailed lists of correspondences can be found in Aleister Crowley's *Liber 777* (published as *The Qabalah of Aleister Crowley*).

Chapter 2

ESSENCE AND QUINTESSENCE: PERFUMERY AND ALCHEMY

This admirable Art, teachest how to make Spirits, and sublime gross Bodies; and how to condense, and make Spirits become gross Bodies: and to draw forth of Plants, Minerals, Stones and Jewels, the Strength of them . . . and to make them more pure . . . and noble . . . and to lift them up as high as Heaven. It is Nature's part to produce things, and give them faculties; but Art may ennoble them.

—John Baptista Porta, *Natural Magick* (1558)

Alchemy is another of the magical arts, representing both a psychological process and a physical process. Both levels are concerned with essence. Paracelsus, a sixteenth-century doctor and theorist, described alchemy as the voluntary action of man in harmony with the involuntary action of nature. The process in the alchemical vessel is analogous to the process of spiritual transformation in the psyche of the alchemist. Two of the main preoccupations of alchemists were the relationship between body and spirit and the perfecting of the soul.

Modern chemistry, metallurgy, and medicine all trace their roots back to the ancient experimental science of alchemy. The art of perfumery also owes a lot to this prototypical science. The physical process of extracting natural perfumes from crude substances has had a long evolution. In this century there has been a revolution in technology. Since volatile oils are found in a wide variety of substances other than flowers, a few new techniques have developed. Though preparation of the raw materials may differ, the three main production techniques are distillation, expression, and extraction.

In removing and concentrating essential oils, the modern perfumer still follows the three main stages of alchemical work: separation, purification, and recombination. This process is expressed in the alchemical axiom, *Solve et coagula*, meaning "Dissolve and combine."

The process of distillation can be seen as a metaphor for human spiritual development. The breaking down (*solve*) and heating of plant materials liberated their essence, or first matter, while *coagula* means to create new substances with additional desirable characteristics. In psychological terms, distillation requires the sacrifice of old notions. It is the breaking down and destruction of outworn or random attitudes that alienate us from the self. The soul, our most characteristic quality, can rise in meditation much as the distillate rises. Through this process the heavenly aspect latent in all earthly things is slowly liberated. Psychologically, *combining* signifies the building of a fully integrated personality. In much the same way, different qualities of volatile oils are married in a mature perfume.

Thus, alchemy may be carried out as either a

physical or mental operation. However, it should not be reduced to only a metaphor of psychological and philosophical transformation. The practice of alchemy always requires experimentation, within the lab or the psyche. The approach to alchemy in Jungian psychology is primarily mental, although it can take physical form. For example, you might ritually act out certain aspects of the Great Work—the process of transforming a base substance to a subtle essence. The interpretation of alchemy as a spontaneous unconscious process comes from a basically mental, or Greek, orientation. (We refer to this type of approach as Greek because the ancient Greeks developed theories—without experimentation—about how the world works.)

The type of alchemy that aims at rejuvenating or preserving the physical body is descended from the physically oriented Egyptian alchemy. The traditions of conscious, inner spiritual alchemy come mainly from the Islamic and oriental philosophies. Using alchemy, the ancients sought to produce medicinal elixirs, essences, and tinctures, as recounted in Junius's *The Practical Handbook of Plant Alchemy*. Alchemy takes its name from an ancient name for Egypt, and this is indeed the land of its origin in the West. This rudimentary experimental science refined mummification with the use of plant substances. Aspects of alchemy spread throughout the Middle East and gained entry to Europe during the Crusades. The Arabs were apparently the first to discover and utilize distillation, or extraction of the spirit of the fragrant substance. The essential oils were equated with the "volatile sulfur," also known as the soul, or Apollo. (For a complete technical description of the extraction of essential oils, see Junius, Chapter 5.)

Arabic alchemy made a great evolutionary leap forward when it was applied by Avicenna or Ibn Sīnā (980–1037). He was primarily a physician, but one who had reputedly mastered Moslem theology and Greek sciences by the time he was sixteen. He is credited with being the first to concentrate *otto*, or attar, the volatile oil of flowers. Prior to that, perfume was extracted largely from gums and barks. A romantic version of the discovery tells how Princess Nourmahal ordered a large tank filled with water and red roses and placed on a barge, so that she could smell the roses as she floated along. As this barge was rowed in the heat of the sun an oil floated on the surface of the water. However the discovery occurred, this early distillation process was simple. The roses were placed in a copper alembic, or vessel, and a fire lit beneath it. Twenty-two pounds of flowers was heated in sixteen gallons of water, and the steam was driven into a vat, where it condensed and ran into a receiving flask. This quantity of flowers produces two one-gallon flasks of rose water. Eight gallons of this rose water are redistilled into a single gallon of distillate. When this cools, the otto rises to the top to be collected with a small ladle shaped like an inverted cone. The oily liquid quickly solidifies, and all excess water is filtered out.

In examining this process, we can create an analogy between the distillation process and psychological and spiritual development. Distillation can be viewed as symbolizing meditation or the striving of the mind up toward the plane of archetypal ideas. Distillation demonstrates the constant interaction of the complementarities, Matter and Spirit. In this case there are four stages to the alchemical process:

1. Spirit attains separate consciousness in matter.
2. After a time Spirit desires identification with the whole universe and sublimates, leaving matter.
3. Matter, however, attracts Spirit back to it, realizing that it is the evolutionary plan of creation to enrich consciousness this way.
4. The two are united again.

This process continues until Spirit has fully absorbed all the lessons of Matter, and at the same time Matter is purged of its grossness. Each distillation represents a step forward. In meditation the consciousness is gradually and painfully expanded by concentration and the striving for right relationship, but it is a very long process.

In alchemical distillation, the crude botanical mass is equivalent to the *prima materia*, or first matter. Psychologically, it is represented by our complexes, or mental hang-ups. It is precisely this lowly, earthy material which is the basis of the work. The next step is to expose it to the heat of the element fire, in the operation known as *calcinatio*. In the developmental process, this fire comes from the frustration of instinctual desires. This frustration leads to spiritual development if one has a viable relation to the self. Even in Homeric Greece, fire was considered a purifier and separator of the soul.

Heat, or fire, causes the essence or soul to free itself from identification with the earthy, gross mass, and it begins to rise. What formerly seemed solid is changed to liquid (*solutio*) and will emerge in a rejuvenated form. In terms of spiritual development, we can remain stuck at a certain stage until we fall in love or develop mystic devotion, when the blocks to further progress are dissolved. This is the work of the element water. We learn to identify with the free-soaring spirit rather than the personality. Thus we push at our limits, gaining access to new states of consciousness. Essence is softened into a liquid, flowing state.

Sublimatio, the operation of air, is an elevating process that transforms a low substance to a higher one by an ascending movement. The steam that contains the volatile oil is driven to the top of the flask, much as the spirit soars free in meditation. Temporarily released from the confines of earthly existence, we are freed from the personality to experience the self's immortality. In terms of psychological development, this means that we learn to see through the concrete, literal aspects of our existence to their inner symbolic meaning. *Sublimatio* leads to the separation of the soul from the body.

Thus, *sublimatio* is an extraction process. It is the process of extracting the transpersonal, objective meaning from our purely subjective interpretations of crises in our lives. Contact with the self releases us from our personal ego attributes. We then gain a living relationship with the archetypal dimension, which was known in the past as paradise or heaven.

Finally, as the steam begins to cool and condense, the volatile essence begins to recoagulate, known in alchemy as *coagulatio*. The distillate takes on a new, highly refined existence, free of dross. The pure essence has been refined and fixed, becoming earthy once again. According to Jung, the process of fixation means the consolidation of feeling as firm convictions and a permanent content.

In psychological development there is both a lesser and a greater *sublimatio*. The greater *sublimatio* leads to union with Godhead. In this instance *coagulatio* has the ultimate meaning of the acquisition of an immortal body. But many rounds of "distillation" are required for this result. Even though one practices mystical meditation, *coagulatio* means that the free spirit is still connected with the limitations of physical life (karma, duties, job, family, and so forth).

The lesser sublimation must always be followed by a descent in which spiritual values are brought back into a well-grounded life-style. In other words, to make insights practical, they must be grounded in daily life. When we view our lives from an elevated spiritual perspective, we are released from the merely personal view. We come to understand that the ups and downs of life have a transcendent, symbolic meaning that was not apparent at first. Another alchemical dictum says, Sublimate the body and coagulate the spirit.

Repeating the upward and downward movement brings refinement through the operation known as *circulatio*, or circulation. It can refer to the repetitions of distillation or to the emotional realization of opposites (ups and downs) leading to their reconciliation. When an essence is thoroughly purified it is fit to combine with others in the operation called *conjunctio*, meaning union, friendship, intimacy, relationship. This marriage or blending of discrete essences reflects the union of the soul with godhead. The result is the quintessence, that which is beyond fire, water, air, and earth.

Returning to the more mundane level of perfumery, we find the old alchemical axiom, *Solve et coagula* still represented in the art as the solvent and fixative. Steam distillation is still the underlying method of processing geranium, lavender, neroli, and other herbs and flowers. Improvement in steam and vacuum stills has improved the product and the economics of extraction considerably.

The process of *expression* is applied almost exclusively to collecting citrus oils. The oil-bearing cells of the peel are broken and the oils sponged up and filtered. The results of this process are poor, so these oils are generally mixed with extracts or with noncitrus oils. The machine process for clarifying oil uses a centrifuge.

Extraction avoids the drawback of applying high temperatures to volatile substances that are destroyed by heat. Extraction can be done with hydrocarbon solvents that are then removed, or by two other means. *Enfleurage* is a means of extracting oil by soaking blossoms in fat. The final method, *maceration*, immerses the flower petals in liquid fat or oils under gentle heat. In both maceration and enfleurage the fat is collected and refreshed with new flowers until the fact is saturated with flower oil. Each method is appropriate for certain types of plants as follows.

Enfleurage: lily of the valley, jasmine, tuberose, orange blossom, jonquil

Maceration: cassie, rose, orange blossom, violet

Solvent extraction: reseda (from *Reseda odorata*) rose, jasmine, jonquil, tuberose, violets, cassie, orange blossom, carnation, mimosa, heliotrope, oakmoss, stock

Different treatments yield slightly differing products even from the same raw material. Because of economics, only jasmine and tuberose are still extracted by enfleurage. Volatile solvents are the best choice for most flowers. Enfleurage was first tried in 1835, by Robiquet, and came into general use around 1890. One of the most frequently used solvents is petroleum ether, but benzene and others also are used.

Chapter 3

INTRODUCTION TO THE MATERIALS OF PERFUMERY

Smell is the sense of the imagination.

—Jean Jacques Rousseau

Perfumery, like magic and alchemy, is both an art and a science. The raw materials of perfumery have a rich and romantic lore spanning the recorded history of mankind. In the earliest days these precious substances were reserved exclusively for use as offerings to the gods, at first chiefly in the form of incense. Then means were found of transforming these wonderful-smelling gums, resins, spices, and flowers into unguents.

These unguents were always offered with other precious gifts at the shrines of the gods. Thousands of years ago the Egyptians were using the "perfume of the gods," frankincense, for temple rites and as a base for perfumes. The earliest recorded mention of this activity comes to us from the fifteenth-century B.C. The tomb of Queen Hatshepsut contains inscriptions that tell of her sending an expedition to the land of Punt (probably the Somali coast) to import frankincense.

The ancients, in particular the Egyptians, created beautiful containers to hold their creations. Archeologists have found ancient perfume bottles made of jade, alabaster, diorite, and other stones. Skilled craftsmen fitted these beautiful containers with amazingly tight stoppers or lids, which effectively preserved the contents. Some of these fabulously carved vases were uncovered with the treasures of Tutankhamen. Even though the tomb dates from about 1350 B.C., the fragrance of these perfumes lingered until they were opened more than 3,000 years later.

The Greeks and Romans also extolled the virtues of the ancient perfume substances. During the Late Bronze Age, circa 1550–1200 B.C., a number of autonomous kingdoms flourished in Greece. This civilization is called Mycenaean. At the town of Pylos, the Mycenaeans developed a highly organized, palace-controlled industry in perfumed oil by the late thirteenth century B.C. They grew and imported ingredients, while the palace subsidized the perfumers and was used for storage of the luxurious finished products. Bronze-Age Pylos used perfumed oils in rituals, most notably those in honor of Potnia and Poseidon. Perfumes were also used as grave gifts, often being placed on the funeral pyre or used to prepare a body for burial. This anointing had a preservative effect.

In the *Iliad*, Homer refers specifically to perfumed oil when Hera prepares to seduce Zeus. Herodotus, Greek Father of History, mentioned the aromatics of Arabia around 450 B.C. He wrote, "The whole country is scented with them and exhales an odor marvelously sweet." At Alexandria, Pliny the Elder described the security on a major processing center: "Good heavens! No vigilance is sufficient to guard the factories. . . . before [the workers] are allowed to leave the premises they have to take off all their clothes. . . ."

Although in ancient times the perfumer was limited to a few natural ingredients, today's aromatic creations can draw upon between 4,000 to 5,000 aromas of organic and synthetic origin. There are a few hundred fragrances of natural origin, but a perfume composer's palette contains about 1,000 to 1,200 materials. Even a skilled professional, however, can only know and effectively use about 400 materials.

Each item in the repertoire of perfumery materials has specific properties that come from their odoriferous molecules or volatile oils. A *property* can be defined as an effect that a material object or substance has on another object or on one or more of the senses of an observer. Clearly, the most important biological property of an odorant is that it has an odor that affects the human sense of smell.

To become adept at using a perfumery material, you must become familiar with the effectiveness or potency of the compound, just as a doctor is familiar with the effectiveness of a drug. If a molecule has an odor, it has a characteristic trait or quality. Describing the characteristic quality is very difficult, but recognizing it by smell is relatively easy. The amount necessary for recognition is called the recognition threshold.

Most of us are aware that olfaction is a complicated phenomenon. In daily life, we rarely encounter a single odorant. Usually, we integrate a multitude of sensations from many stimuli to form a composite sensation. The constituents of perfumes may be well over the threshold concentrations. As concentrations exceed the threshold values, the sensations evoked may not be the same as those near thresholds. Vapor pressures vary considerably, by several orders of magnitude, with different media. Some molecules are very unstable and decompose in a matter of minutes, while others are quite tenacious.

The creative art of the perfumer lies not so much in the making, or distilling, of simple odors (which generally consist of the solution of an attar or essential oil extracted from a plant substance in alcohol), as in the unique blends of several ingredients. These blended perfumes are known as bouquets.

In beginning to formulate our own bouquets, we can take note of the practices of master perfumers. Computer statistics of daily use of aromatic raw materials show that while 600 items are used regularly, fifty of these basics make up 80% of the volume used annually. These fifty are the most widely available and should form the basis for the beginner's palette. Also, select no more than 400 aromatic raw materials in total, either synthetic or natural.

Humans cannot assimilate knowledge of thousands of odoriferous substances, including the quality, durability, and intensity of each. To master perfume composition, even on an amateur level, it is wise to limit yourself and achieve intimate familiarity with a few substances in the initial phases of your practice. Each fragrance is like a musical note separated from its melody. It is accurate or true to its own quality but, combined in a melody line (bouquet), it takes on new life.

A famous French perfumer, Pierre Dhumez, has spoken of blending perfumes in the following manner:

> To make a perfume is to find a harmony of three or four dominant "bodies" that you smell in your mind. You have an inspiration for a mixture of those three or four bodies, not more. And they will release themselves in such a way that when you have combined the "corps" in the proportions by which you have been inspired when you were in a tranquil, happy state of mind, you will not be able to distinguish one odor from the other among your basic raw materials. It is a perfectly balanced mixture which smells as a separate entity from the odor of each of the three or four bodies you have chosen—and in so doing you will have created the "woman." After that you have to enhance her—make her more beauti-

Exercise C HOW TO WEAR PERFUME

Commercial perfumes smell different on different people, so it is important to know what type of fragrance you are seeking, and how to buy and wear it for the effect you want.

Mass-marketed fragrances are composed of three elements: a solvent, the fragrance materials, and a fixative to harmonize the rates of evaporation of the various ingredients. This maintains a more consistent smell in the perfume as it dries out.

Different products contain varying ratios of essential oils to alcohol. A product with more alcohol is a more fleeting fragrance. Perfume (parfum) is the strongest and most expensive fragrance you can buy. Its ratio of essence to alcohol is quite high.

Next in order of strength comes eau de parfum, with more alcohol, then eau de toilette, and finally cologne. It is interesting to note that contemporary perfumes are at least twice as strong as those of the last century. They must compete with environmental pollutants and a plethora of cheap fragrances in common household items. Use unscented hairspray, deodorant, and detergents.

Your skin characteristics play a role in how perfume reacts with your chemistry. People with oily skin absorb and retain perfume molecules more easily. The fragrance is fat-soluble and oily skin slows down the evaporation process. If you have dry skin, buy a more concentrated form of essence for a longer-lasting scent. In fact, anyone can maximize the life of their fragrance application by "layering" it on. Since scented products come in so many different forms, you can use the whole line.

Begin by bathing with a scented soap. Moisturize with a body lotion using your chosen fragrance while you are still wet from the bath. Splash on eau de toilette freely. Then, to finish up, apply perfume (or bath oil, undiluted) on your pulse points at the temples, behind the ears, on your wrists, and behind your knees.

If you prefer a subtle, light scent use only toilet waters and colognes. Europeans, Britons, and the French, in particular, scorn the use of strong perfumes, which are considered vulgar. Yet Americans consume large quantities of these so-called "stinker" perfumes, while Germans prefer very expensive perfumes that give an aura of good taste and personal wealth.

If you live or work in an air-conditioned building, be aware that indoor atmosphere's stronger vapor pressure removes the aura of the perfume from around your body. In this case, wear your stronger scents during the day rather than just at night.

Heavy oriental scents or ambers are best worn in fall and winter. Pack them away in spring and switch to lighter, more buoyant scents. Pick one signature fragrance and wear it all the time, or choose many fragrances to go with your moods.

Biological factors may influence how your perfumes smell at different times. A weight loss or diet change may affect them; for example, changing from a high-fat to a low-fat diet. Antibiotics can change your natural skin bacteria, which in turn affects the chemical reactions of your fragrance and your skin.

---

ful; do her hair, select her dress, her lipstick, her eye liner, her hat, her wrap—and that is a perfume.

A perfume (known more commonly as a scent in Great Britain) is much more than a pleasant smell; it is a unique sensation produced by a harmonious blend of materials, sometimes as many as a hundred different odors. The perfume gives a single pleasant impression, like the chords of a musical composition blend to form a beautiful symphony. In a bouquet, each odor must be brought to a certain standard of strength, so that no single scent overpowers the others.

NATURAL RAW MATERIALS

The most useful and least expensive form of perfumery ingredients are known as essential oils. These are isolates distilled from natural sources such as odoriferous gums and resins, fresh or dried leaves, buds, flowers, berries, fruits, nuts, beans, pods, seeds, roots, rhizomes, twigs, and wood itself. Other sources include barks, mosses, lichens, and balsamic or resinous exudations. Maurer provides a useful, if not exhaustive, classification of these natural sources.

1. *Flowering plants, shrubs and trees:* Cananga odorata, carnation, cassie, hyacinth, jasmine, jonquil, mimosa, narcissus, neroli, reseda, rose, tuberose, violet, ylang-ylang.
2. *Leaf oils:* Bay, cinnamon, cedar, eucalyptus, patchouli, petitgrain (*citrus aurantium*), wintergreen.
3. *Wood oils:* Amyris, balsamifera (West Indian rosewood), birch, bois de rose (rose oil steam distilled from wood), cade oil (juniper tar), camphor, cedar, guaiac, laurel, lináloe, santal (sandalwood), sassafras.
4. *Leaves, needles, and twigs:* The pines—abies, silver, sylvestris, sibirica, and so forth, and cajeput, cassia, cedar, cypress.
5. *Bark oils:* Birch, cassia, cascarilla, cinnamon.
6. *Fresh fruit oils, cold expressed:* Almond, bergamot, citron, grapefruit, lemon, lime, mandarin orange, and tangerine.
7. *Grass oils:* Citronella, gingergrass (*Cymbopogon martini*, var. *sofia*), lemongrass, palmarosa (*Cymbopogon martini*, var. *motia*).
8. *Seed oils:* Ambrette (from *Hibiscus abalmoschus*), angelica, cardamon, carrot, croton, cumin, dill, mustard, parsley.
9. *Dried leaf oils:* Cherry laurel, eucalyptus, niaouli (*Melaleuca veridiflora*), patchouli.
10. *Dried fruit oils:* Anise, coriander, fennel, juniper, nutmeg.
11. *Dried buds and berries:* Clove, cubeb, juniper, pimento.
12. *Balsam oils:* Balm of Gilead, copaiba, labdanum, Peru, tolu.
13. *Gums:* Elemi, galbanum, mastic, myrrh, olibanum, opopanax (*Commiphora erythrea*), storax.
14. *Roots and rhizomes:* Angelica, calamus, costus (root of *Saussurea lappa*), ginger, orris, valerian, vetiver.
15. *Herb oils:* Basil, chamomile, clary, dill, estragon (tarragon oil), fennel, geranium, lavandin (*Lavandula hybrida*), lavender, lovage, marjoram, origanum (from *Thymus canatus*), parsley, pennyroyal, peppermint, rosemary, rue, sage, spearmint, spike lavender, tansy, thyme, verbena, wormseed, and wormwood.

Also of major consideration are those perfumery products derived from animal sources, the most widely used being ambergris, musk, and civet.

The main drawback of these classifications is that they offer little that can be used by the beginner in actual perfume compounding. Still, it is useful to learn the sources from which materials are derived. More important—since most perfumes are based on a floral foundation—is an organized palette accommodating a minimum number of the floral types. From these, balanced floral components can be created upon which to build further. Maurer also offers a table that can be used "as a perfumer's equivalent of the artist's shade-card," showing how you can combine blossom fragrances to make perfumes (see Table 1). Working regularly with this table will teach you the nature and strength of odor of these natural aromatics.

By trying every possible combination of these basic groups you will develop a feel for what will and will not work. You can re-create such well-known bouquets as jasmine-neroli-rose or rose-jasmine-carnation. Other classics which come from this "palette" of essential oils include lily of the valley-jasmine-carnation, carnation-jasmine-violet, ylang-ylang-carnation-jasmine, and gardenia-lavender-carnation. Odors of the same group blend well together, but those blends combining groups may be more interesting. Any of these basic combinations can be enhanced or accented with more complex florals or other botanical oils.

Forming such bouquets is much the same as working on scales for the aspiring musician: it is a necessary step toward developing your skill in this creative field. With a firsthand knowledge of the basics, you can begin experimenting by adding more and more subtle accents to your original blends. These are the essentials of compounding perfumes.

There are many other natural raw materials, too

TABLE 1 An Arrangement of Blossom Fragrances and Perfume Types

PRIME ODORS Group 1	PRIME ODORS Group 2	SIMPLE EXOTIC FLORALS Group 3
1. Jasmine	6. Violet	11. Gardenia
2. Neroli	7. Lily of the valley	12. Hyacinth
3. Rose	8. Lilac	13. Mimosa
4. Carnation	9. Lavender	14. Heliotrope
5. Clover blossom	10. Verbena	15. Ylang-ylang

numerous to describe in this volume. You can find further information in *Perfumes and Their Production*, Edward S. Maurer (1958) and *Natural Perfume Materials*, translated by Edward Sagarin from the French in 1949. In the magical employment of perfumes, it is good to work with essential oils in their pure form, without cutting them with alcohols. Their scent is then released by the gentle heat of the body, rather than by the evaporation of alcohol. Also, they exert a subtle influence by actually being absorbed into the body to some extent. Using natural rather than synthetic products may be more aesthetically pleasing.

SYNTHETIC MATERIALS

The floral kingdom contains more than 4,000 scented substances that perfumers can use to compose scents, but many are expensive to harvest and yield little oil upon processing. As replacements for these hard-to-get essences, a wide variety of synthetic perfumery substances have become available in the twentieth century. While the natural products might seem more aesthetically pleasing, our experience has shown that the psychological effects of the synthetics serve much the same purpose as their natural counterparts. In some cases, they are preferable—for example, substituting synthetic musks or ambergris for those taken from animals, rather than supporting the killing of endangered species.

Synthetics are disdained by some as lacking the warmth of natural substances. This is easily corrected by the addition of small amounts of essential oils to round out a fragrance. One of the most lastingly popular perfumes in the world, Chanel No. 5, was one of the first to include synthetic ingredients. Its introduction by Coty, in 1927, was soon followed by that of L'Aimant and Arpege. Synthetics brought fabulous perfume creations within the budgets of the masses.

In the 1980s, the designer fragrance market is getting crowded. Different types of scents are popular at different times, but women's perfumes are a perennial favorite. One of the most successful lately has been Giorgio. Also popular have been the oriental types, like Opium, Poison, Cinnabar, and Shalimar. The trend toward Romanticism may see the resurgence of more floral types, like Estee Lauder's Beautiful. In its July 27, 1987, issue *Chemical Marketing Reporter* noted that "the trend is fresh, floral and outdoorsy. Most of the new aroma chemicals reflect this trend, although musk replacements are also still being developed."

In the 1930s, men's colognes became popular. The images portrayed in the 1960s' advertisements for such fragrances as Brute and Hai Karate were very macho. Now the ads are suggestive: male models are cast in sexy poses, in part because women were found to buy 75 percent of men's fragrances.

In these days of mass merchandising, we all long to be unique. If you find a perfume you especially like, make a similar blend, but add your own unique touch and make it even better—for you or a loved one. You may ask, "Where do I start?" A little research will give you leads. Gaborit's *The Essences and Their Bottles* (1985), for example, contains a table listing the primary components of 200 of the world's great perfumes.

Today's sophisticated perfumes are so subtle in composition that changing the formula just a little will alter the final result dramatically. Making such small changes is one way to gain the knowledge of master perfumers and build your own skill. Don't be afraid to experiment with synthetics once you have a basic knowledge of essential oils. Today, more than two-thirds of the materials used in perfumery are man-made.

Even an introduction to the synthetics would require another volume. Some of the basic synthetics are ionone (derived from the Greek *ion*, from which the violet took its name), and eugenol and iso-eugenol, which are carnationlike. Terpineol reproduces the odor of purple lilac, while styrolyl acetate has an odor resembling gardenia flowers. Hydroxycitronellal enabled the creation of synthetic lily of the valley. Linalyl acetate has a sharp, lemonlike smell. Geraniol has a rose scent.

CONCLUSION

In providing a rudimentary knowledge of perfumery materials, our goal is to free you from the primitive sense of smell. As a beginner, you will find many scents you like and don't like. Approach your art with imagination, rather than biases, because the many modifications scents undergo in combination alters their character dramatically. An essence that seems overwhelming or sickening straight from the bottle can provide just the right accent in the proper amount.

Never depend on one particular supplier. Many suppliers of different sizes offer similar materials under different names for widely varying prices. The larger perfume houses with better-quality product often have very costly minimum purchases. You will have to shop around and be somewhat flexible to get the items you want at an affordable price.

Odor classification systems are provided only to give a solid foundation for your further exploration of the magical realm of psychosensory evocation. We are attempting here to lead you, as a beginner, to a dialogue with the perfume materials and even more toward learning to speak the language of perfumes. The multitude of luxurious essences can be described in terms of dimension (a flat, linear odor), mass (heavy), volume (rich, full), tactility (rough), taste (bitter, sour), temperament (violent, nervous, youthful, sparkling), or eroticism (warm, sensual). Perfumes can be described by words derived from flowers, fruits, resins, woods, herbs, and chemicals.

Some descriptive responses to scents are cultural in origin. The French, famous for their acute olfactory discrimination, have over 500 words in their language directly related to the sense of smell. Many impressions depend on various human reactions and associations shaped by the traditions, customs, conventions, and prejudices of any given culture. The Japanese, for example, find the odor of civet offensive because it reminds them of decaying flesh; they prefer ambergris, which is somewhat reminiscent of fish. Natives of Africa and the Middle East favor spicy, warm, strong, and heavy scents, as do the East Indians. Perfumes of this type are generally characterized as oriental. Scandinavians prefer light, floral fragrances—perhaps to remind them of spring during endless winters. The Chinese favor the fragrant blossoms of peach, magnolia, jonquil, and jasmine.

We are all influenced to some extent by olfactive stereotypes, sometimes on a deeply subconscious level. A geranium-cinnamon combination tends to suggest the smell of soap. Chrysanthemum means death. Violet is often interpreted as cheapness, unlike rose and jasmine, or it may remind you of an old aunt you never really cared for. We come to associate certain odors with unpleasant as well as pleasant situations, thus our likes and dislikes are built up over the years at the subconscious level. Patchouli, once considered a vulgar odor in England, came to be one of the signature scents of the flower children, along with the standard sandalwood.

Bear in mind that in perfumery as in other arts, style is an important component. It is the special touch that makes a perfume composition more than the sum of its less sophisticated substances. All great perfumes radiate their special style, and each perfumer has a unique style. In music, painting, and literature, the notes, colors and words are the same, but the development and use of individual style allows for an unlimited variety of artistic productions and differing interpretations of the same theme.

You can approach perfume composition visually and rhythmically, almost like an olfactory ballet. Your choices of quantity, quality, and combination of fragrances directly influence the way they are harmonized. A simple style, an unsophisticated formulation, yields a simple, unsophisticated perfume with the advantage of clarity and spontaneity. Complex formulations will create complex perfumes that unfold in softer, less abrupt rhythms.

When composing a perfume, always write down the ingredients you use as you add them—do not trust your memory, or you may lose the formula of your most delightful creation. An effective, cheap way to test your creations is to use coffee filters cut up into long, thin strips. Test your creation at every stage of development—allow time for the different scents to blend and mature. Smell the test strip when you first mix them, then test a few hours later and compare. Smell the same strips later, even the next day; This will also show you the staying power or tenacity of the scent. Be sure to label the test strips with some code and the date. To get the full effect always test the scent from the strip waved in the air, rather than from the bottle.

You may be a visual person, who likes to use symbols for various scents when working them out on paper. One simple form of writing down a perfume (olfactive writing) links a simple graphic design to a scent. You can work out your own system according to the feeling you get from the various fragrances. These forms can be abstract or symbolic, but they add to your fluency in the language of perfumes. The shapes you use will probably stay consistent for some period of time, but they may evolve over longer periods.

Using your imagination in the creation of perfumes means linking together bits of olfactory information that have never been associated before. This quest is a daily search, the attempt to duplicate or capture the essence of some attractive smell from daily life: the garden at dusk, damp earth after a rain, tree bark, the forest, a wood fire. You cannot create without inspiration. As you turn your attention more and more toward scent, you become aware of the keen variety of different odors and learn to appreciate them in a new way, much like learning to appreciate fine wines.

Perfume is a language, the language of fragrances. As a form of communication it ranges from single odors to simple formulations into sophisticated compositions. When purchasing a perfume for themselves or others, most people tend to use just a few vague words to describe what they are seeking. Without better descriptors, it is difficult to know what they mean. If someone asks for a "soft" perfume, does that mean sweetly soft? Vanilla soft? Musk soft? Soft as opposed to strong? A "cool" perfume might mean citrus cool, peppermint cool, lilac cool, a cool touch, or feeling cool.

What is needed is a more common language among producers and users of perfumes to fill the requirements and needs of one another. Perhaps this is even more important in the magical employment of perfumes, where small suppliers fill the requests of a variety of customers. Since the substances are serving an important symbolic purpose, it is important that the client get what he or she asks for. A little basic education in the perfumery art goes a long way toward achieving this goal.

Chapter 4

THE LANGUAGE OF PERFUME

*Love, that is crimson, sumptuous, sick
with perfume,
No other words but words of love, no
other thought but love.*

—Walt Whitman

Odor classification is one of the first major considerations in developing your fundamental knowledge of perfume blending. This was not such a monumental problem before the introduction of synthetics. To simplify this problem it is best to investigate first the commoner essential oils and flower extracts.

There are three main odor classifications used as standards: Rimmel, Piesse, and Crocker and Henderson. That of Crocker and Henderson is the most simplistic, reducing the elements of sensation that make up all odors to just four kinds. These four types are related to four kinds of olfactory nerves, and their elementary odor sensations are: fragrant or sweet, acid or sour, burnt or empyreumatic, and caprylic or oenanthic. This classification is hardly useful for blending purposes.

Rimmel's system is more useful, being based on eighteen distinct types of similar or compatible fragrances. Knowledge of odors belonging to the same class is useful even if somewhat static in application. Rimmel's classification, from his *Book of Perfumes*, appears in Table 2.

Charles H. Piesse, in *The Art of Perfumery*, gives perhaps the most inventive and fluid classifications by comparing odors with sounds. He claims that scents, like sounds, appear to influence the olfactory nerves in certain definite degrees. He draws an analogy between octaves of odors and octaves in music, and says that certain odors coincide, blending into chords.

Piesse positioned the odors in correspondence with musical notes according to the scent's effect on his olfactory sense. To use his schema for creating a bouquet, shown in Table 3, choose the odors that chord together and your perfume will be harmonious. Steer clear of discords. For example, almond, heliotrope, vanilla, and clematis blend together; citron, lemon, orange peel, and verbena form a higher octave. Semiodors, such as rose and rose-geranium, are equated with half notes.

FORMS OF PERFUMERY INGREDIENTS

The main forms of directly usable perfumery ingredients include concretes, absolutes, resin absolutes, resinoids, and essential oils. As stated before, essential oils are generally the least expensive and most widely available of the prepared fragrance sub-

TABLE 2 Rimmel's Classification System

CLASSES	TYPES	ODORS BELONGING TO THE SAME CLASS
Almondy	Bitter almond	Laurels, peach kernels, mirbane
Amber	Ambergris	Oakmoss
Anise	Aniseed	Badiane, caraway, dill, fennel, coriander
Balsamic	Vanilla	Peru, tolu, benzoin, storax, tonka
Camphoraceous	Camphor	Rosemary, patchouli
Caryophyllaceous	Clove	Carnation, clove pink
Citrine	Lemon	Bergamot, orange, cedrat, limes
Fruity	Pear	Apple, pineapple, quince
Jasmine	Jasmine	Lily of the valley
Lavender	Lavender	Spike, thyme, serpolet, marjoram
Minty	Peppermint	Spearmint, balm, rue, sage
Musky	Musk	Civet, ambrette seed, musk plant
Orange flower	Neroli	Acacia, syringa, orange leaves
Rosaceous	Rose	Geranium, sweetbrier, rhodium, rosewood
Sandal	Sandalwood	Vetiver, cedarwood
Spicy	Cinnamon	Cassia, nutmeg, mace, pimiento
Tuberose	Tuberose	Lily, jonquil, narcissus, hyacinth
Violet	Violet	Cassie, orris-root, mignonette

stances. You will probably deal with them most often, but it is useful to know about other concentrations of the ingredients.

CONCRETES, as the name suggests, are the densest, least refined manufactured product. They are usually solid, waxy, noncrystalline masses, which develop crystals of almost pure aroma constituents upon standing. Concretes are water-insoluble extracts prepared from natural materials by using hydrocarbon-type solvents. They are prepared exclusively from materials of botanical origin such as barks, flowers, herbs, leaves, and roots. Concretes differ from resinoids by being extracted from formerly live tissue, not plant exudations. All plant tissues, including fiber and cellulose, have been eliminated. The result is only partially soluble in perfume oils, but it contains a large amount of alcohol-soluble absolute.

ABSOLUTES make up from 20% to 80% of concretes, with a common content of 50%. They are highly concentrated fragrance products that are entirely alcohol-soluble extracts of concretes or related fat-soluble or waxy materials. Usually they are extracted under gentle heat, frequently more than once, to exhaust the concrete. All alcohol-insoluble substances are cold-filtered out (sometimes a centrifuge is used) before evaporation of the solvent. Absolutes are generally quite expensive, requiring large amounts of costly botanicals to produce.

Occasionally, the name absolute is also given to the alcohol-soluble fractions of resinoids. This product differs slightly from the so-called alcohol resinoid, known commercially as resin absolute. An absolute is produced from a raw material extracted with petroleum ether to produce a resinoid, which in turn is extracted with alcohol to yield the absolute. This is done, for example, with labdanum. Petroleum ether extractions of natural gum resins and oleoresins yield results suitable for further purification into absolutes.

RESIN ABSOLUTES, or alcohol-resinoids, are produced by direct alcohol extraction of such natural raw materials as gum resins and oleoresins. Heated alcohol is used to extract the resin absolute from raw botanical material, plant material, or gummy exudations. It is then distilled under vacuum pressure to recover all the alcohol. Examples include oakmoss resin, labdanum resin absolute, and orris resin.

TABLE 3 The Range of Odors as Arranged by Piesse

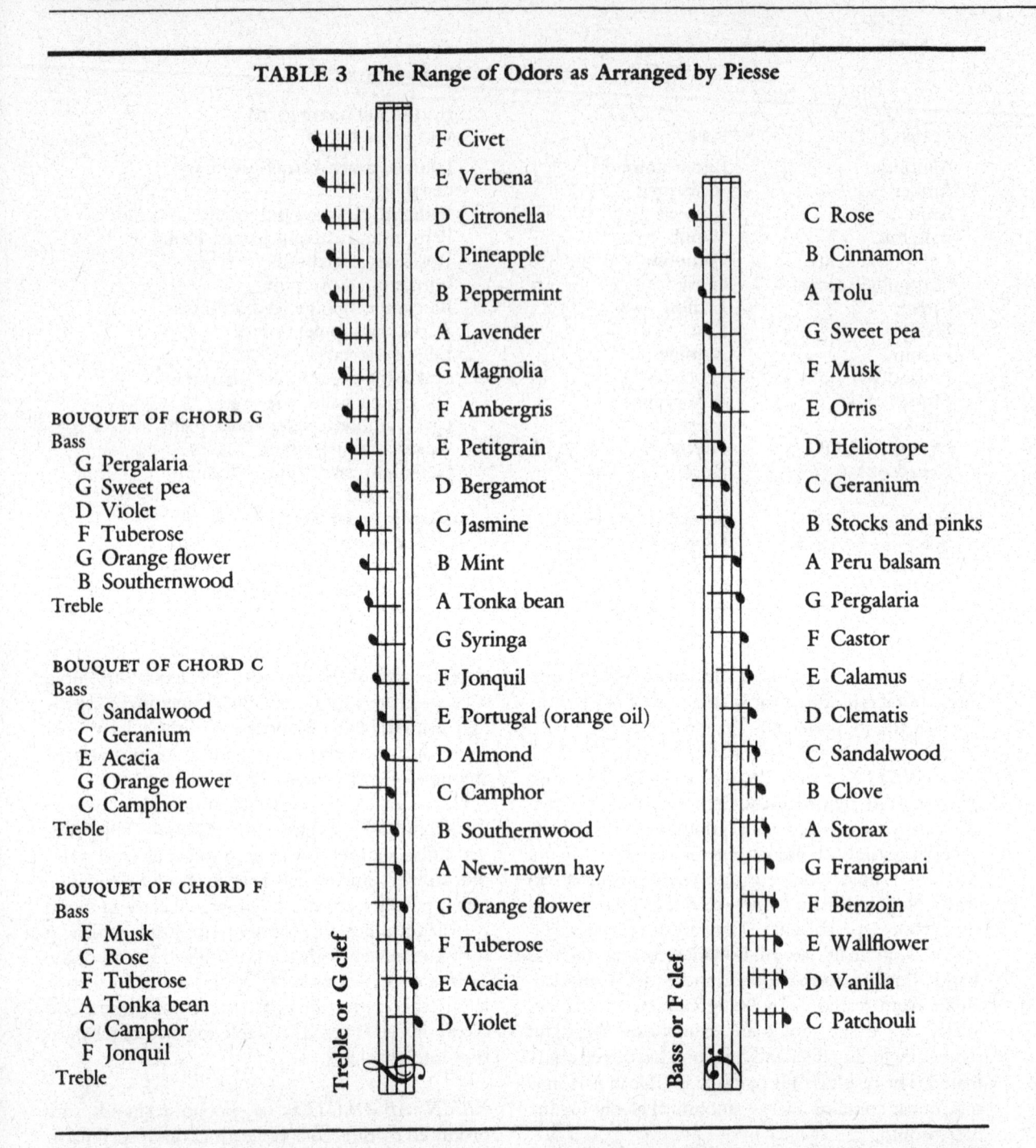

BOUQUET OF CHORD G
Bass
  G Pergalaria
  G Sweet pea
  D Violet
  F Tuberose
  G Orange flower
  B Southernwood
Treble

BOUQUET OF CHORD C
Bass
  C Sandalwood
  C Geranium
  E Acacia
  G Orange flower
  C Camphor
Treble

BOUQUET OF CHORD F
Bass
  F Musk
  C Rose
  F Tuberose
  A Tonka bean
  C Camphor
  F Jonquil
Treble

Treble or G clef:
- F Civet
- E Verbena
- D Citronella
- C Pineapple
- B Peppermint
- A Lavender
- G Magnolia
- F Ambergris
- E Petitgrain
- D Bergamot
- C Jasmine
- B Mint
- A Tonka bean
- G Syringa
- F Jonquil
- E Portugal (orange oil)
- D Almond
- C Camphor
- B Southernwood
- A New-mown hay
- G Orange flower
- F Tuberose
- E Acacia
- D Violet

Bass or F clef:
- C Rose
- B Cinnamon
- A Tolu
- G Sweet pea
- F Musk
- E Orris
- D Heliotrope
- C Geranium
- B Stocks and pinks
- A Peru balsam
- G Pergalaria
- F Castor
- E Calamus
- D Clematis
- C Sandalwood
- B Clove
- A Storax
- G Frangipani
- F Benzoin
- E Wallflower
- D Vanilla
- C Patchouli

RESINOIDS are the viscous liquid, semisolid, or solid perfumery products extracted from resins, gum resins, and oleoresins with hydrocarbon solvents. Unlike concretes, resinoids are produced from non-cellular organic material not once-living plant tissue. Resinous materials include balsams and admixtures of gums and resins. The finished product contains all the hydrocarbon-soluble material, including the resins, but the solvent is removed. This usually leaves a homogeneous mass of noncrystalline, or amorphous, nature composed mainly of rosin acids, rosin acid anhydrides, sesquiterpenes,

Exercise D EXPERIMENT WITH SCENT

Essential oils form the basis for all perfumes. Their concentration and accompanying ingredients determine the type of product. Begin by experimenting with very simple combinations like rose-lavender, rose-cinnamon with a little musk, or jasmine and neroli (orange blossom). Also try musk or ambergris with rose. "Greener" scents can be made with patchouli, lavender, rose, and civet, musk, or ambergris. A good male fragrance can be made from balsam, cedar, or sandalwood mixed with musk and cinnamon. "Cut" these simple blends with alcohol to create a variety of products. Use tiny perfumer's funnels and glass eyedroppers, but wash them scrupulously to avoid contaminating your inventory.

ESSENCE

Pure essential oils are known as essences. Their blends are called perfumes. Blends of pure essences are rare, since most commercial perfumes contain only about 15%–30% essential oil cut with alcohol. Pure essences have more oils to interact with oils in your skin; they are tenacious and with proper fixation last from 4–6 hours. Wear them on pulse points at ankles, knees, wrists, cleavage, and throat.

EAU DE TOILETTE (EAU DE PARFUM)

Eau de Toilette has a significantly lower percentage of essential oils than an essence. Containing only 10%–15% essence, it can be applied more liberally, but it lasts only 2–4 hours.

COLOGNE

Cologne contains even more alcohol than eau de toilette. Splash it on freely, but it lasts only 2 hours. The basic formula for cologne is one part oil, six parts perfume diluent or vodka, and one part fixative. Try this recipe from aromatherapy:

rosemary oil	5 parts
neroli oil	20 parts
lemon oil	75 parts
lavender oil	5 parts
bergamot	220 parts
alcohol 90%	5,000 parts

EDIBLE MASSAGE OILS

These contain 1%–3%, or 20–30 drops, of pure essential oils per ounce (30 gm). Try the ratio of ¼ oz. of fragrant oil to 4 oz. of an unscented oil such as wheatgerm or apricot oil. A blend for Relaxing Oil has 10 parts geranium, 5 parts lavender, 4 parts marjoram. Aphrodisiac oil can be made from 7 parts bergamot, 3 parts rose, 3 parts jasmine, and 7 parts sandalwood.

BATH OIL

These contain a nice percentage of essential oils diluted with a fixed oil of weak scent. Use 5–10 drops per tub of water. Experiment with this simple formula:

ylang-ylang oil	2 drops
sandalwood oil	8 drops
jasmine oil	2 drops

BATH POWDER

Mix a few drops of the fragrance blend of choice with cornstarch or arrowroot.

SKIN FRESHENER

For an after-bath splash try one part oil, ten parts diluent or vodka, one part fixative.

AIR FRESHENER

A mixture of 12 parts bergamot, 2 parts eucalyptus, and 4 parts juniper heated with a light bulb is refreshing.

essential oils, plant colors, and waxes. Extra essential oil is neither added nor removed during refining of resinoids. Oleo-gum resins include myrrh, galbanum, and olibanum, the natural resin of which has been made soluble in perfume materials by removing the water-soluble gum.

Prepared oleoresins have the oily and resinous materials extracted from them with fat solvents such as hexane, ether, and alcohol. The solvent is then removed under vacuum pressure, leaving behind a viscous, semisolid extract known as the oleoresin, the most concentrated liquid form of botanical material.

Pure resins, the natural plant exudates, have little direct value. They rarely occur in nature without being mixed with volatile oils and gums, so in commerce the term *resin* is used for all the resinous materials.

ESSENTIAL OILS, also known as essences, ethereal oils, or volatile oils, are the odorous principles found in various plant parts. They are termed volatile because they readily evaporate when exposed to the air at ordinary temperatures. They represent the essences of the fragrant chemicals produced by a plant. They are usually complex admixtures of hydrocarbons, alcohols, ketones, esters, phenols, acids, ethers, aldehydes, oxides, and sulphur compounds.

Essential oils are generally processed out by steam distillation, solvent extraction, or expression. The resulting volatile oils are generally pale or colorless when fresh, but they may oxidize and resinify with age, becoming darker. Always store your oils in a cool, dry place in amber glass containers to protect them from light. The stoppers should fit very tightly on bottles kept as full as possible. As the bottle empties, transfer the oil to a smaller bottle for longest shelf life.

As scented oils of plants, volatile oils differ widely in their chemical constitution, but they have a great number of physical properties in common. Essential oils are:

1. Volatile at ordinary room temperatures
2. Can be steam-distilled at ordinary pressures
3. Do not leave permanent grease stains on paper
4. Do not contain glycerides and therefore do not form soaps with alkalies
5. Do not become rancid on exposure to air but tend to resinify when oxidized
6. Mix freely in any proportion with chloroform, ether, or absolute alcohol

The chemical characteristics of volatile oils are often a valuable diagnostic property (i.e., to test for adulteration).

PERFUMERY NOTES

We have already seen how fragrances can be classified according to a musical analogy. Carrying that analogy further, we present the concepts of top, middle, and base notes. Most perfumes include the three notes to produce a smooth, harmonious odor.

Top notes are the volatile, fleeting essences. They are the first to be smelled at the threshold of recognition, and the first to evaporate away, leaving the other tones to predominate. Some examples are lemon, lavender, and anise oils. The intermediate class, or middle notes, volatilize more slowly; they include the oils of rose, neroli, and thyme. Base notes are those products with the lowest volatility and highest tenacity. They are also described as *fixatives* because of their ability to add staying power to the perfume composition. The most notable examples are the animal products ambergris, musk, and civet (and their synthetic counterparts), although there are botanical fixatives as well.

First, it is of great importance to create the right atmosphere for your study of perfume on the blotters. A constant room temperature and relative humidity are highly desirable, if possible. Temperatures of 20°–27°C (68°–80°F) are considered most conducive, even down to 17°C (62°–63°F) in a highly professional setting. Relative humidity should be maintained between 45% and 50%. Excessively low or high humidity is unfavorable to smelling. One quick trick to remember if your conditions are less than ideal: exhale hot, moist breath from your nostrils or mouth onto the dry, previously dipped blotter to reactivate the scent by steam distillation and enhance a weak-smelling fragrance.

To gain familiarity with notes, you will need to run several blotter tests. From coffee filters, cut smelling strips about ¼ in. (6 mm) wide and 5–6 inches long (12–14 cm). Mark your strip clearly with the name or number of your sample, then dip it about 2 inches into the essential oil. Study the odor immediately, after a few minutes, in half an hour, in several hours, the next morning, until there is no odor left. By taking notes, you will learn its properties and be on your way to becoming an amateur "nose." You'll learn that the lighter notes quickly rise high on the blotter, while larger molecules remain at the end where it was dipped.

TOP NOTES—known as *la note de depart* because they are the first note to volatilize as the bottle is opened or scent is applied—should be studied repeatedly, because they last such a short time. Since it is the first impression of odor, it can be characteristic of an essential oil and difficult to duplicate in a synthetic. Since top notes cannot be studied at length, you may want to refresh your scent memory on various topnote oils at different times in your perfumery career.

MIDDLE NOTES or *body notes* reveal the overall characteristic odor of the oil on the blotter. They are slightly less characteristic than the top note but easier to reproduce with artificial products. Note the length of time each of your oils maintain its body note on the blotter in a loose-leaf notebook.

BASE NOTES, also known as dry-out notes, are just as important as the top note. The dry-out reveals not only the fixative effect of the oil but can reveal adulterations of your essential oils. Study base notes repeatedly and carefully, noting your observations for future use. The dry-out may take from one to several hours or days, depending on the oil. Many oils, such as patchouli, vetiver, civet, and everlasting, require at least 24 hours of observation. The body note may persist to the end, but the topnote will not, except in the very powerful angelica oil.

The dry-out reveals a scent's tenacity. Tenacity lends a fixative quality to a perfume composition. Fixatives as a class usually have a high boiling point and high molecular weight; this retards their evaporation and helps slow the loss of more volatile components in solution with them. We will return to fixatives and their use shortly.

FIXATION AND BLENDING

Fixation is one of the most important factors in perfume composition for the public, because they demand products that have staying power. As early as 370 B.C., Theophrastus is recorded as saying, "Those perfumes whose scent is strongest get the best hold on the skin, head, and other parts of the body, and last the longest time. . . . the stronger a perfume is the longer it lasts." Four hundred years later Pliny spoke of resins and gums as fixators: "The very highest recommendation of them is, that when a female passes by, the odor which precedes her may possibly attract the attention of those even who till then are intent upon something else . . . for the person who carries the perfume about with him is not the one, after all, who smells it."

FIXATIVES are used primarily for slowing down the rate of evaporation of the volatile portions of a perfume. The fixative is a less evanescent substance, which also creates a body on which to build the perfume. At the same time, they must allow the predominating note of the fragrance to be retained. In other words, they equalize the different rates of evaporation of the constituents.

There are four main types of fixatives, and a perfume material may belong to one or more of them. They include the following:

1. *The True Fixatives:* These retard evaporation by the physical effect of adsorption due to their densely packed molecules. Example: benzoin.
2. *The Arbitrary Fixatives:* These hold their note throughout all phases of drying out but do not influence evaporation rates of other ingredients. Example: oakmoss.
3. *The Exalting Fixatives:* These bases carry odor but also improve and fortify the other ingredients with their synergistic effect. They give a perfume wearability, tenacity, and luxurious

diffusiveness. Because of their strength, only traces of them are required. Examples: musk, civet.

4. *The So-Called Fixatives:* These odorless substances have high boiling points that increase the boiling point of the entire perfume. As stabilizers, they "steal" some of the qualities of the perfume, but they also balance and conceal minor errors. Example: amyris oil.

Fixatives also may be classified by their source: animal, vegetable, or synthetic. Another system uses the headings pleasantly aromatic, disagreeable, and neutral. In the first category are benzoin, olibanum, tolu, musk, ambergris, sandalwood, clary sage, benzyl iso-eugenol, vanillin, coumarin, and Peru balsam. Some of the disagreeable substances are asafetida, valerian, civet, skatole, castor, and indole. Benzyl benzoate, ethyl phthalate, and glyceryl acetate are neutral fixatives.

Fixation is a tricky process, sometimes requiring several stages. It is fairly easy to add small increments of fixative to a sophisticated blend with good results. The trick is to blend fixators into imitations of floral scents. Here, some blend better than others. Orris oleoresin can be used in violet, for example, benzyl iso-eugenol or vanillin in carnation and clove pink, indole in jasmine, and patchouli in white rose.

PREFIXATION is the deodorization of alcohol into an aromatic spirit, which blends more easily into the final product. The easiest way to do this is to add to the alcohol a resin extract (benzoin R, for example) that is similar in scent to the result you want.

BLENDING is the addition of modifying fixators during production. Violet perfumes harmonize with sandalwood, costus, ylang-ylang, and orris; lily of the valley accommodates bois de rose, ylang-ylang, and hydroxy-citronellal; carnation takes heliotropin, iso-eugenol, and benzyl iso-eugenol. For most florals, you are safe with coumarin, vanillin, and heliotropin, while chemicals such as methyl naphthyl ketone or dimethyl hydroquinone will add a *de luxe* aura.

FINAL FIXATION is a delicate operation that adds life to your creation. A touch of animal fixative will soften synthetics. Sweetness may be increased

---

TABLE 4 Classification of Fixators

1. ESSENTIAL OILS

Basil	Nutmeg[1]
Bois de rose	Origanum
Cananga	Patchouli
Cassia	Peru
Cedarwood	Saffron
Clove	Salvia sclarea
Coriander	Santal
Costus	Sassafras
Cumin	Spikenard
Cypress	Sumbul
Guaiac-wood	Tarragon
Iris	Thuja
Linaloe	Thyme
Mace	Valerian
Marjoram	Vetiver
Myrtle	Ylang-ylang

2. BALSAMS, GUMS, OLEORESINS, ETC.

Ambrette	Male fern
Ammoniacum	Mastic
Angelica	Moss—Corsican
Asafetida	Myrrh
Benzoin	Oakmoss
Chamomile	Olibanum
Cascarilla	Opoponax
Costus	Patchouli
Clove	Peru
Copaiba	Sandarac
Elemi	Santal
Galbanum	Sumbul
Geranium	Storax
Ginger	Tolu
Iris	Tonka beans
Juniper	Vanilla
Labdanum	Vetiver

[1]Expressed
Source: Poucher, W. A., and Howard, G. M., *Perfumes, Cosmetics and Soaps,* Vols I–III.

---

with bois de rose, bergamot, or verbena. A touch of natural absolute will enliven a flowery note with jasmine, rose, or mimosa. Just strive for complete harmony among your ingredients. Good animal fixatives, or high-quality synthetic analogs, are one of your most indispensable assets. Musk xylol, ketone and ambrette, exaltone and exaltolide, indole and skatole, and artificial ambers are passable substitutes for animal products, especially when combined with high-quality essential oils and absolutes.

Ambergris is best for eau de cologne, while large proportions of a musk-civet mixture are good for oriental blends. Vegetable fixators, such as myrrh, frankincense, and spikenard are wonderful for equalizing varying rates of evaporation. Tenacious essential oil fixatives include angelica, clary sage, orris, patchouli, santal, and vetiver, all of which have a high boiling point. Vetiver and patchouli also work for oriental bases. Clary sage is unparalleled as a base for synthetic florals and as a blender and fixer in alcoholic perfumes and eau de cologne.

Resin odors, or *clairs* (also known as R), are easy to use, especially in nonalcoholic perfumes, where they may constitute as much as 30 percent of the product. Those with strong odors can be used as a small percentage of the whole, say, 5 to 10 percent. Benzoin is weaker, while labdanum and olibanum are strong. Others include storax, oakmoss, orris, Peru, and copaiba.

Artificial fixatives include coumarin, vanillin, heliotropin, musk Baur (one of the earliest patented musk formulations), phenylacetic acid (honey and civet), benzoic acid, cinnamic acid, amyl benzoate, benzophenone, benzylidene acetone, benzyl iso-eugenol, skatole, and the aldehydes, such as cyclamen, phenylacetic, decyl, undecyl, and methyl nonylacetic. A good rule of thumb with synthetic fixators is to add them carefully with an equal weight of balsam or gum resin to balance out any hint of chemical.

FAMILIES OF ODORS

Perfumes for women are classified by families of odors, while perfumes for men are not. These families include (1), floral, (2) green (pine, herbs, camphor, mint), (3) citrus, (bergamot, neroli, petitgrain), (4) oriental, (5) chypre, (6) aldehydic, (7) leather/animal, and (8) fougere (fern).

Floral is a nonspecific term and can mean anything from a single note of floral essence to over a hundred notes in a floral bouquet. Some well-known florals include Joy, White Shoulders, My Sin, Arpege, and Quelques Fleurs. Green scents range from fresh and sporty to richer balsamic scents. Examples include Chanel No. 19, Lauren by Ralph Lauren, and Geoffrey Beene. Citrus scents are well represented in colognes. Oriental blends are uninhibitedly erotic and have a pronounced, heavy sweetness with balsamic or woody notes. They include Youth Dew, Tabu, Shalimar (a mild amber), Cinnabar and Opium (semiflowered ambers), Dioressence, and Chantilly.

Aldehydics are frequently called modern blends. They are imaginative and combine real essential oils with complex synthetics. They are characterized by rosy-floral odors or floral-woody-powdery notes. Famous aldehydic types are Chanel No. 5, Je Reviens, Arpege, Jontue, and Chamade. Chypre blends are complex and earthy, combining moss, woods, flowers, and sometimes citrus. Examples include Miss Dior, Forever Krystle, Ma Griffe, Intimate, and Ciao.

Leather/animal scents are aromatic, heady, and sensual. Leather is pungent and smoky with a light sweetness. Examples include many of the musk oils, Cachet, and English Leather. Fougere notes are fresh and aromatic, using lavender for emphasis. Contrast is added with dry tones of oakmoss and rare woods. Fougere Royal (Houbigant) is a premier example; it was the first to make use of synthetic coumarin. Ambush is another example. While the fern and leather families are not subdivided, other families are. Florals include soliflore (single floral note), floral bouquet, green flowered, aldehydic flowered, and fruity woody flowered types. Chypres include aldehydic flowered, fruity chypre, leather chypre, and green chypre blends. Orientals are sometimes called amber. They include woody flowered amber, spicy flowered amber, mild amber, semiflowered amber, and amber aldehydic.

These various classifications of scent show their affinities by smell. Other affinities can be determined by examining their use in magic, ritual, and the qabalistic system.

Perfume Magic

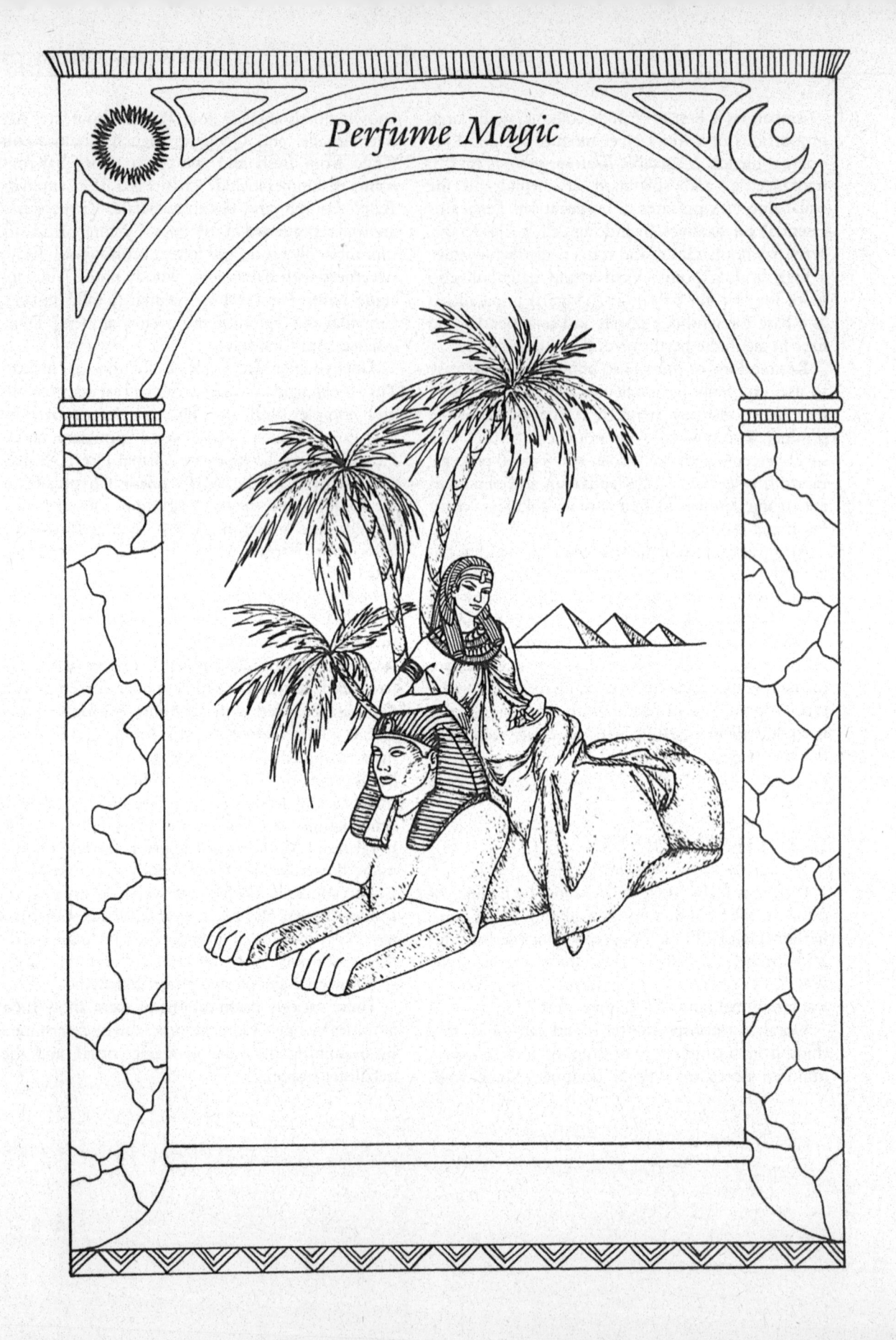

Chapter 5

THE ESSENCE OF QABALA

Magical practices are the projections of psychic events . . . by means of these concrete performances the attention, or better said, the interest, is brought back to an inner sacred domain which is the source and goal of the soul. This inner domain contains the unity of life and consciousness which, though once possessed, has been lost and must now be found again.

—C.G. Jung, *Secret of the Golden Flower*

The practical application of the Qabala in magic involves artistic employment of correspondences—the linkages of colors, scents, tones, astrological signs, and tarot attributions as well as the qualities of gods and goddesses. When you assemble all the components of a given archetypal force in your working area, they exert a symphonic effect on your psyche. Since scent is so closely linked to memory, using particular scents primarily in ritual circumstances makes it easy to recapture the feeling tone of past workings.

Odors arouse our personal memories as well as those from our deeper mind, the collective unconscious. Through the years, fragrances have been associated with cosmic forces and their corresponding gods. For example, many people are familiar with the odor of sanctity produced by frankincense burning in Christian churches. Frankincense has a long history of use in cults of solar gods such as Osiris and Apollo. Originally, inspiration implied breathing in a sacred scent along with the force it represented. Scents help create the archetypal atmosphere during ritual; it only takes one whiff of a scent to which your subconscious is conditioned to put you in the frame of mind you have cultivated using ritual.

Scents can also be used outside of ritual as a means of balancing the personality or emotional nature. You might find out which elements are missing from your astrological chart, choose the corresponding scents from the qabalistic tables, and wear those scents to round out your self-expression. You could also formulate your own astrological scent using the fragrances of your sun, moon, and rising signs, or other important aspects of your chart.

Psychology shows us that there are innumerable archetypes, but those on the Tree of Life have been shown by tradition and practice to be those most relevant to man's spiritual growth. Likewise, there are over 5,000 ingredients in the perfumery art. Just as perfume displays the essence of the flower, so the soul or spirit of a person can be seen as the essence of his or her body. Certain scents continue to be valued beyond monetary considerations and exert an ageless appeal on the psyche.

Perfumes and incenses have been employed in rites for both their physical and metaphysical effects. They serve three purposes in ritual:

1. They provide a material vehicle of fragrant smoke for the manifesting energy (that is,

they create a surface on which to visualize).
2. They are offered as a costly sacrifice.
3. Their intoxicant effect penetrates the consciousness.

Aromatherapy—therapy by the use of essential oils—has recently become popular. The qabalistic system can also be employed therapeutically: scents can be used to heal faulty relationships to the gods. The Greek word *therapeuein*, "to heal," originally meant "to serve the gods." Thus, all healing takes place in a sacred context. Healing also connotes becoming whole. If you want to round out your psychological and sensual experience, use scents to stimulate the desired qualities. For example, Aphrodite = aesthetic appreciation = benzoin, rose, or sandalwood; Hermes = intellect = storax, amber, spikenard.

Another way of using scents in Qabala relates them to letters (see Figure 1 in the preface). Each letter of the Hebrew alphabet corresponds to a path on the Tree of Life. Each path has a fragrance, therefore each letter has an odor. (The corresponding English letters are given in the appendix.) It is possible therefore to blend scents that literally spell name or words—god-names, names of angels and intelligences, or of your significant others. The scent helps you get you on the right wavelength. Some blends are seductive, some are exciting, yet others are tranquilizing.

In Magick, the practice of practical Qabala, perhaps more than in any other area where scents are employed, it is most desirable to have the highest-quality ingredients, as well as a working knowledge of their source and use. The more you experiment with blending, the more highly developed your nose will become. Practice and experience will work harmoniously with intuition to guide you into creating truly heavenly aromas for yourself.

The qabalistic correspondences are broken into two main groups. The first group represents the numbers of the Spheres, 1 through 10. The second group represents the Paths, 11 through 32. Each number of each group has innumerable correspondences, but those most relevant to our purpose include the Qabala and Tarot attribution, the astrological correspondence, tone, color, and scent (see Table 5). Each sphere of the Tree of Life represents a discrete state of consciousness. The paths are the means of transition from one state to another. Each

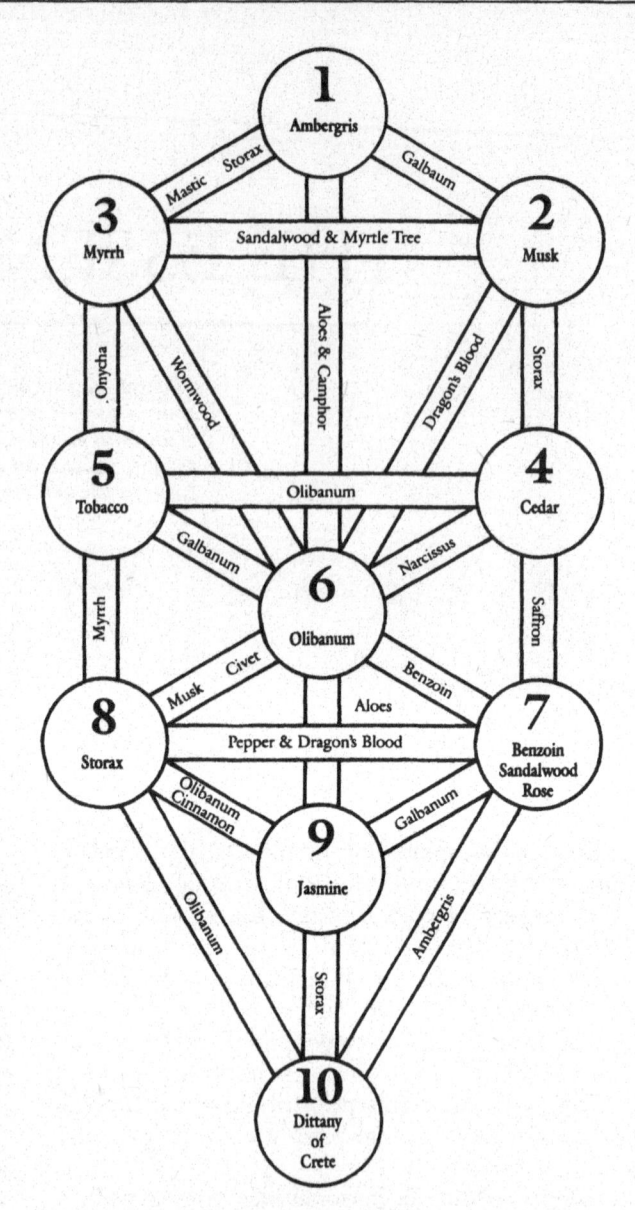

Perfumes on the Tree of Life

has a set of symbols used to stimulate the imagination toward the desired condition during ritual. These are the basics for creating and re-creating a structured sensory experience. They are used to invoke the force they represent. With the scents, one literally inhales the essence of the god or quality.

TABLE 5 Correspondences

KEY	ASTROLOGY	NAME	TONE	COLOR	SCENTS
Essence of the Spheres					
1	Origin	Kether		White	Ambergris
2	Zodiac	Chokmah		Gray	Musk
3	Saturn	Binah		Black	Myrrh, civet, madonna lily
4	Jupiter	Chesed		Blue	Cedar, oakmoss
5	Mars	Geburah		Red	Tobacco, leather
6	Sun	Tiphareth		Yellow	Olibanum (frankincense), angelica
7	Venus	Netzach		Green	Benzoin, rose, sandalwood
8	Mercury	Hod		Orange	Storax, amber, spikenard
9	Moon	Yesod		Violet	Jasmine, ginseng, orris
10	Earth	Malkuth		Tertiaries	Dittany of Crete, poppy, patchouli
Essence of the Paths					
11	Air	Fool	E	Yellow	Galbanum
12	Mercury	Magician	E	Orange	Storax, mastic
13	Moon	Priestess	G#	Violet	Camphor, aloes
14	Venus	Empress	F#	Green	Sandalwood, myrtle
15	Aries	Emperor	C	Scarlet	Dragon's blood
16	Taurus	Hierophant	C#	Red-Orange	Storax
17	Gemini	Lovers	D	Orange	Wormwood, orchid
18	Cancer	Chariot	D#	Orange-Yellow	Onycha, lotus, labdanum
19	Leo	Strength	E#	Yellow	Olibanum (frankincense)
20	Virgo	Hermit	F	Yellow-Green	Narcissus
21	Jupiter	Wh. of Fortune	A#	Blue	Saffron
22	Libra	Adjustment	F#	Green	Galbanum
23	Water	Hanged Man	G#	Blue	Onycha, myrrh
24	Scorpio	Death	G	Blue-Green	Benzoin, opopanax
25	Sagittarius	Art	G#	Blue	Lign-aloes
26	Capricorn	The Devil	A	Violet	Musk, civet
27	Mars	Tower	C	Red	Pepper, dragon's blood
28	Aquarius	The Star	A#	Purple	Galbanum
29	Pisces	The Moon	B	Magenta	Ambergris, lily, honeysuckle, violet
30	Sun	The Sun	D	Yellow	Olibanum, cinnamon
31	Fire	The Aeon	C	Red	Olibanum
32	Saturn	Universe	A	Indigo	Storax, castoreum, cypress

\# = sharp note

Exercise E Consecrated Oils

Consecration carries the connotation of making sacred. Any oil you have purchased will hardly have its proper effect unless you charge it symbolically with specific virtues. Thus charged, or consecrated, it is devoted, in your mind, to a particular result.

When dedicating any new oil or perfume blend to its new purpose, first perform the Banishing. If you have a good, multipurpose anointing oil, like oil of abramelin or tetragrammaton oil, you can anoint the bottle of the new oil with an appropriate symbol, such as its astrological correlate.

Open the bottle and volatize a portion of the oil, either by wearing it or heating it gently. As you smell its fragrance, contemplate the key qualities you now consciously associate with it. See yourself embodying those traits. See and hear how others respond to you when you evoke these resources. Imagine how you will feel when these qualities are totally integrated into your personality. This creates a holistic association between the fragrance and the state of consciousness you wish to anchor.

In de Laurence's classic magical work, *The Greater Key of Solomon*, an exorcism for purifying sacred incenses and perfumes is given.

O God of Abraham, God of Isaac, God of Jacob, deign to bless this odoriferous incense/perfume so that it may receive strength, virtue and power to attract the Good Spirits, and to banish and cause to retire all hostile Phantoms. Through Thee, O Most Holy Adonai, Who livest and reignest unto the Ages of the Ages. Amen. I exorcise thee, O Spirit impure and unclean, thou who art a hostile Phantom, in the Name of God, that thou quit this incense/perfume, thou and all thy deceits, that it may be consecrated and sanctified in the name of God Almighty. May the Holy Spirit of God grant protection and virtue unto those who use it; and may the hostile and Evil Spirit and Phantom never be able to enter therein, through the Ineffable Name of God Almighty. Amen.

O Lord, deign to bless and sanctify this sacred essence so that it may be a remedy unto mankind for the health of the body and of the soul, through the Invocation of Thy Holy Name. May all Creatures who receive the odor of this incense and of these spices receive health of body and of soul, through Him Who hath formed the Ages. Amen.

The fragrance bottle is then sprinkled with holy water, wrapped in an appropriately colored silk, and placed in a cool, dark place for future use. Crowley called consecration "the active dedication of a thing to a single purpose." The single purpose of this scent is now to anchor those qualities symbolized by its station on the Tree of Life. Doing a banishing over your perfumes prevents their use for any other purpose, but they are inert until you consecrate them to a particular goal. As a secular or earthly substance it must be purified by the element Water, banished by the element Air, and consecrated by Fire, as symbolized by the holy oil. Then the fragrance forms a magical link with the archetypal force it represents. Imagination is reality and in the imagination, symbols are not abstract forms but living realities.

One might wonder why scents don't affect us more overtly if they function at a subliminal level. They do not automatically evoke those characteristic traits because they are not employed in a meaningful context. Using scents in a magical operation is like using a gun to fire bullets instead of merely throwing them. The penetrative power is exponentially magnified.

The Essences

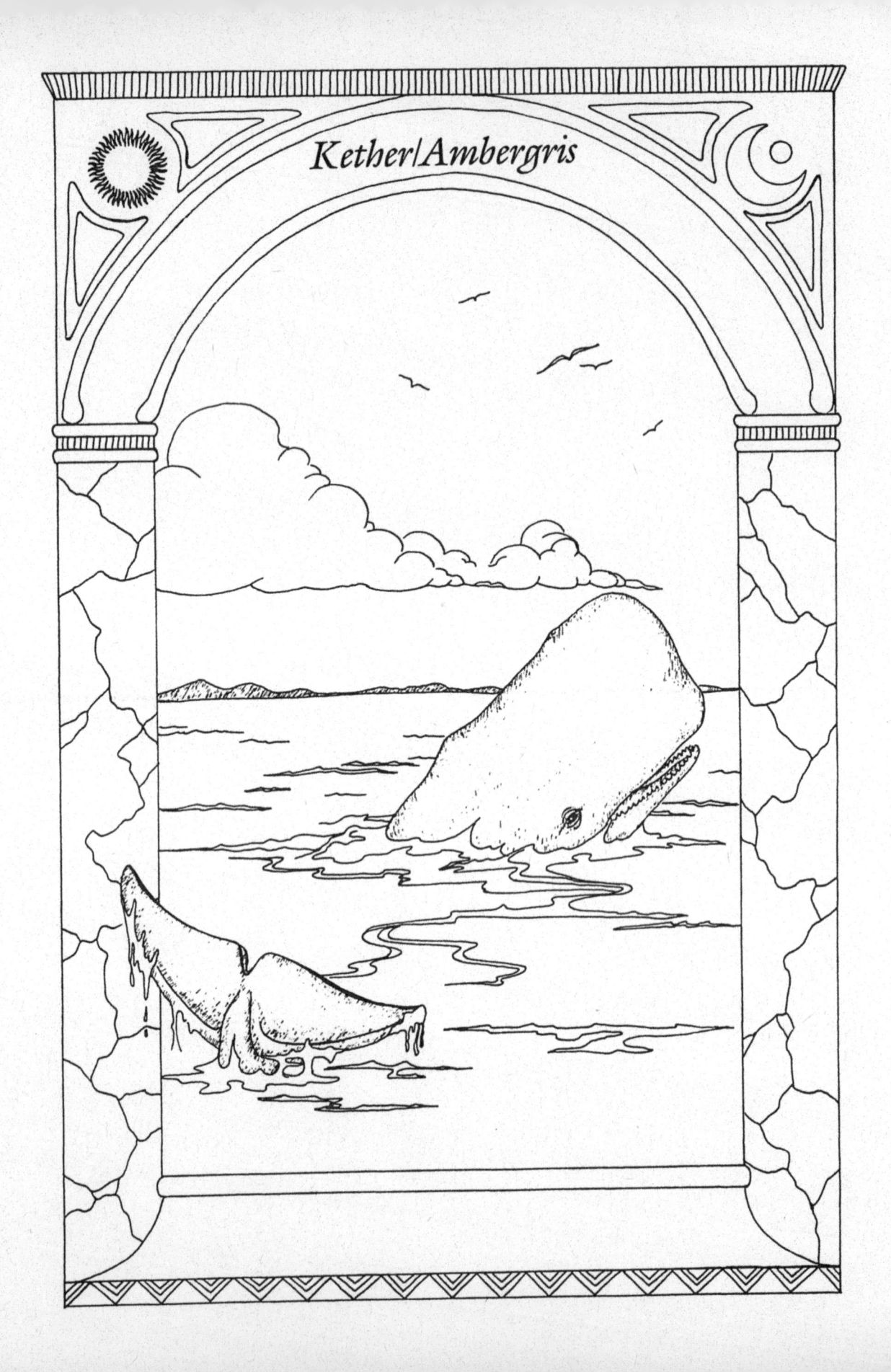

Kether/Ambergris

> *Ambergris has comparatively little perfume of its own, but it has a virtue of bringing out the best of any other with which it may be mixed. In the same way, Kether cannot be said to have any intrinsic qualities, but its influence brings out the highest faculties of those ideas which it illuminates.*
>
> —Aleister Crowley, *777*

1. KETHER = AMBERGRIS

QABALA

Kether, according to qabalistic doctrine, is the source of All, including that which is beyond manifestation. In human terms, it represents the reunion of a pure soul with Godhead. Kether symbolizes that source beyond the creator God, or Universal Mind. Universal Mind is limited to the Causal Plane, below the Abyss on the Tree of Life. Kether is known as the Crown, and symbolizes the crown-chakra. Thus, wearing the scent of Kether can be seen as a psychosensory stimulation of your crown center—the top psychic center above the head in yogic philosophy. Stabilizing consciousness at this center is the goal of human spiritual evolution. Of course, wearing the scent won't take the place of the inner work of meditation. Rather, it functions as a mnemonic device, directing your attention and contemplation toward spiritual development. Your personality affirms its identification with spirit by seeking the light above your head. Keywords, or qualities we seek to stimulate with this scent, include completion, devotion, eternity, peace, perfection, restoration, and unity.

DESCRIPTION

Reflecting its attribution to Kether, ambergris is considered one of the most valuable materials used in perfumery. It comes from the sperm whale, or cachalot, and it is now boycotted voluntarily by the perfume trade for ecological reasons. Ambergris is produced largely by the male of the species after feeding on squid or cuttlefish (*Elodone moschata*), which has an indigestible beak. The whale's irritated digestive system surrounds the offending substance with a pathological growth, ambergris. The whole mass is passed or vomited out. Ambergris is an amorphous lump of no single size or weight. Color varies from black and brown to grey or chalky white. It floats because of its waxy spongy texture.

It takes an expert to identify good ambergris. It has a specific gravity of 0.900 and melts at fairly low temperatures. The best ambergris is light grey or white, having been exposed to sun and sea. It is so rare that the largest find of top-quality, pure white ambergris was recorded at 20 ounces. The darker the mass, the less it is worth because of contaminants. The heart or core of a lump is the purest, most desirable portion. True ambergris softens at 60°C and readily liquifies at higher temperatures. It is soluble in ether as well as oils and consists of about 80 percent ambrein, an odorous substance found in the cuttlefish beaks subjected to bacterial action.

GEOGRAPHIC LOCATION

Where whales are found, or as flotsam washed ashore. Main finds in the past were from Africa, the Persian Gulf, and the Austroasiatic Pacific. In more recent times, finds are made at whaling stations in the intestines of dissected sperm whales.

HISTORY

The history of ambergris is long, as it has been highly prized for many centuries. For most of that time no one was sure just where ambergris originated. It was valued as an aphrodisiac and as a fragrance and fixative. Legends and conjecture surrounded its procurement. Ambergris has been an important trade item since at least A.D. 1000 when the Arabs spread its romance to many nations.

A New Zealander was reported to have found a lump weighing 42 pounds. Earlier finds averaged between 150–270 pounds, with the largest being 926 pounds, marketed in 1953. Large finds are more rare nowadays and often are covered with dirt and other waste material. High-quality, relatively clean parcels of 15–70 lbs. are found in the intestines of the whales, while larger chunks come from the stomach. Ambrein, the crystalline, odorous material, is the "glue" that holds the mass together.

The process of extracting ambergris has evolved over the last two centuries. French perfumers originally ground it with sugar candy, mixed it with rose spirits, and set it in the sun to mature. Other chemists used some musk, cinnamon, lemon, orange, and lavender. The earliest perfume manual in English, by Charles Lillie (1822), gives a recipe mixing 1½ ounces of ambergris with 30 grains of musk and 20 grains of civet. This was added to sugar and solvent and placed in horse dung for 21 days to create spirit of ambergris.

SCENT AND APPEARANCE

The odor of ambergris is difficult to define. It has a low-intensity odor, with the fixative quality of lifting or "exalting" other odorants. This effect is strong when combined with musk or civet, as well as floral or aldehydic notes.

The smell ambergris is described as being earthy, musty, musky, and reminiscent of the sea. It is a discrete, smooth, and pervasive odor. Some of the most luxurious perfumes contain ambergris.

From ecological concern, many prefer to use the excellent synthetic ambergris products now available. Advantages include cost, availability, and consistent quality. Although their odors differ slightly from real ambergris, they are in no way inferior in their psychological effect. Still, some magical purists will insist on using the real thing. If your style of working demands the natural ingredient, be ready to pay through the nose to get it!

Typical extractions of ambergris vary in color and odor. Powdered ambergris is mixed with alcohol and agitated by machine for several days at a temperature of 25°–30°C. Bottles are then occasionally shaken as the contents mature. Before use, the product is filtered for usable extract. One must be an expert to evaluate the results.

Synthetic ambers are offered in solid, semisolid, and liquid forms, blended with other scents. The main constituent, methyl nonyl acetic aldehyde, is also sold as amber aldehyde. There are three main classes of amber notes: (1) Fixateur 404 (Firmenich), (2) Amrophore and Grisambrol (Firmenich) and Ambrarome (Synarome), and (3) reproductions based on labdanum.

The first and finest of these has a dry, woody, earthy, natural odor that builds over time and is tenacious. Grisambrol almost duplicates natural ambergris and so must be used in minute quantities. A little of it mixed with musk and civet would make an excellent Kether scent and would represent the entire Supernal Triad, composed of spheres 1 through 3 and representing the most spiritual aspects of existence. The labdanum-based synthetics are mixed with musk, civet, castor, and modifiers of jasmine, rose, patchouli, clary sage, and so forth to soften the chemical odor.

BLENDING

Ambergris is the slowest to evaporate of all perfumery materials. Due to cost and availability, use of this extract is confined to preparation of the finest perfumes. Its delicate odor does not compete with delicate florals. No synthetic can compare with the natural product in mellowing perfumes, and the amount used depends on the style of the perfumer.

Modern tincture of ambergris is prepared by dissolving 2% to 3% concentration in 95% alcohol. This mix is stirred by machine for at least three months, neutralized with ammonia, and filtered. The longer the period of maceration and aging, the better the result—providing the original substance is of good quality.

Tincture of ambergris (3%) can be replaced by much less expensive synthetics with excellent results. A good substitute is 3% tincture of ambergris synthetique (Givauden). Another substance to use with great restraint on account of its strength is Fixateur

404 (Firmenich). Dosages of 0.1% to 0.2% of a perfume concentrate may be two or three times too strong.

You can mix your own reproduction of ambergris, using labdanum resin, olibanum resin, Liquidambar, Storax resin, benzoin resin absolute, tolu and Peru balsams, oakmoss absolute, clary sage oil, sandalwood oil, patchouli oil, vetiver oil, cypress and costus oils, and civet. Chaulmoogra oil, cold-pressed from seeds of *Taraktogenos kurzii* King, yields a tincture that simulates ambergris on the human skin. It imparts warmth and sensuality to perfumes.

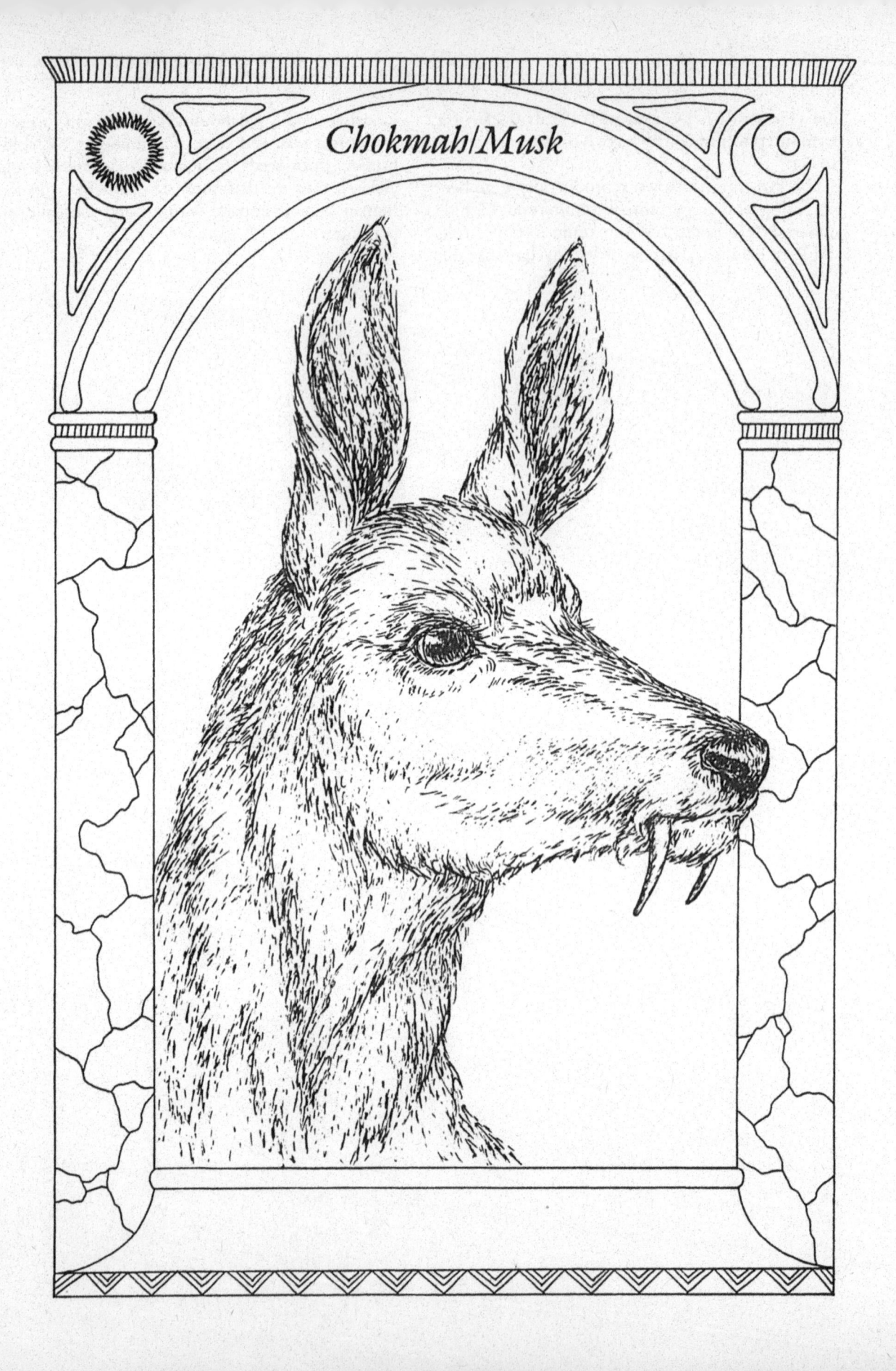

Chokmah/Musk

THE ESSENCE OF THE QABALA 41

> *The ground of this enchanted place is composed of pure wheaten flour mixed with* musk *and saffron: its stones are pearls and hyacinths, and its palaces built of gold and silver . . . The houris are made of pure musk.*
>
> —Prophet Mohammed, describing paradise in the Koran

2. CHOKMAH = MUSK

QABALA

Sphere 2, Chokmah represents the principle of divine Ideal Wisdom. We experience it as libido, dynamic outpouring energy. It corresponds with the third eye, or ajna chakra, therefore it is associated with meditation. In Oriental systems this energy of the masculine principal is termed *yang*. We can tap this divine dynamo through the magical employment of musk, which represents the subliminal, psychological aspect of this sphere.

In the lore of perfumery, ambergris, musk, and civet—the animal substances—attract the most attention. Perhaps this reflects their attribution to the Supernal Triad, the highest valued state of consciousness. These scents have an archetypal appeal to the deepest level of our psyche, and we can attune to their quality by using them. These animal perfumes contain unique, surprising details. Keywords for Chokmah include consciousness, creative genius, libido, logos, pure spirit, spiritual energy, transformation.

DESCRIPTION

Musk comes from the male musk deer, *Moschus moschiferus*, and other *Moschus* species. Once again, for economic reasons and because of cruelty to the musk deer, synthetics are dominating the market in terms of volume if not quality. Musk scents both light and heavy were popular in the commercial market from the late 1970s into the early 1980s. The musk deer habitat ranges from Siberia and Korea through China and Tibet to the Himalayas, but the finest musk comes from Tibet. The deer has no antlers, but has elongated canine teeth which protrude downward like fangs or tusks. With big ears and small tails, the deer's greyish-brown hair is long, coarse, and brittle. Musk is produced in a gland, or musk pod, situated in the sheath of the male sex organ. The gland measures 2 to 3 inches in diameter and weighs about one ounce when dry.

These nocturnal animals do not herd together, which makes them difficult to hunt and capture. Inaccessible terrain and the deer's acute hearing make it even harder, not to mention altitudes in excess of 8,000 feet. Legend says they were captured when the hunter played a haunting melody on a flute, attracting them out of the dense brush. Nets or traps in the pathways proved ineffective; hunters resorted to driving them into blocked-up ravines. Does and young animals were killed indiscriminately. Glands from bucks were removed and dried in the sun, on a hot stove, or by immersion in hot oil. Hunting musk deer is now banned.

Musk is shipped in the pod, semidried (15% moisture). Most is consumed in China, where it is esteemed as a medicine. Sometimes unscrupulous dealers adulterate their product. To prevent this, the pods are protected by customs seals. Musk grains form the raw material for preparation of musk tincture or extracts. Up to 65% to 75% of the weight of the pod consists of grains. A lower-grade product is extracted from the lining of the pod, which is known as the blueskin.

Tonquin musk from Tibet, Szechwan, and the Vietnamese mountain areas accounts for about 85% of all imports. It comes in "caddies," containers of about 21 oz. Cabardine musk comes from Mongolia and Siberia and is next in grade. Yunnan musk comes in a different shaped-pod, called *pig-faced*.

The small pods of Assam and Nepal are not highly esteemed.

GEOGRAPHIC LOCATION

The musk deer inhabits a wide range in central Asia but is hunted primarily in Himalaya-Altai, Tibet, southern China, and northern India. Inferior species inhabit the Szechwan-Tibetan border, Yunnan, and other parts of China.

HISTORY

Musk is among the animal scents the origin of which was enveloped in mystery and legend for centuries. First used in India, China, and Persia, it probably came to Europe through Arabia. We find it mentioned in A.D. 1189 as part of a tribute sent to Saladin by the Holy Roman Emperor. As late as the seventeenth century in Europe, musk was erroneously thought to come from cats, like civet.

Musk first appears in English literature in 1398, when a manuscript speaks of "boxes made to kepe in muske and other spicery." In 1400, Lanfranc cites its use in medicine, and in 1570, Hayluyt's "Voyages" mentioned it as one of the trade goods of black Africans.

Musk deer were considered royal property in India. Tartar tribes bartered to get access to either hunting districts or pods, which they promptly adulterated with dried blood or lead shot. In the Middle East, musk was valued as an aphrodisiac as well as for its alleged medicinal properties. It was for some time included in the British *Pharmacopoeia*.

Modern witchcraft employs musk as an aphrodisiac. Prepare the potion while your attention is riveted on the image of your beloved. Grind together a pinch of ambergris, half a pinch of musk, and 12 apple seeds. Add 7 ounces of red wine and boil till three-quarters evaporated and bottle. Add sparingly to consommé, fruit juices, or cocktails.

SCENT AND APPEARANCE

Musk, as a natural raw material, is the most indispensable article used in perfumery, esteemed for both its subtleness and diffusive power. Perfumes without it are often accused of lacking life, which can be seen as reflective of Chokmah, the life principle. The characteristic scent has given rise to the adjective *musky*.

A fixative, musk also enhances the diffusive properties of perfumes and adds lift. The odor is sweet, smooth, and mildly animal, and persistent; it has a mellowing, sustaining, and diffusing result in perfume blends. Ambrette seed oil, Chaulmoogra oil, orris, and vanilla tincture all share something of the musk scent.

Musk includes about 0.5% to 2% of a dark brown oil containing muscone, the odorant. Other constituents are cholesterol, fat, wax, albumins, and ammonia. It has the chemical property of reducing the vapor pressure of other chemicals by physical attraction. Musk is so strong it rapidly fatigues the olfactory nerves. Fifty percent of pure musk is soluble in water, while 10% to 20% dissolves in alcohol.

MUSK TINCTURE is prepared to suit the demands of the user. The resinoid, called resin absolute, is prepared by extraction and is free of most of the fatty insoluble matter of the crude grains. It is pale brown or dark amber, the typical color of aged musk.

MUSK ABSOLUTE is made from alcohol extraction of resinoid, which creates a very viscous, dark brown liquid of intense musk odor. It is among the costliest of perfume materials. You might want to keep it in your safe deposit box. Tincture is easier to handle, with less risk of using too much.

SYNTHETIC musks come from at least six different structural classes of chemical compounds that possess the odor of musk. They include the macrocyclic, benzene, nitro, steroid, indane, and tetrahydronaphthalene (Tetralin) types. Members of all classes, including muscone, have been synthesized, for example, synthetic nitro musks include musk ketone, musk xylene, and musk ambrette. Plants with musk-like odors include angelica seed (*Angelica archangelica*), abelmosk (*Hibiscus moschatus*), musk mallow (*Malva moschata*), musk rose (*Rosa moschata*), musk thistle (*Carduus nutans*), and musk orchis (*Herminium monorchis*).

BLENDING

Natural musk is generally prepared for use in perfumes by making a tincture of 3% grain in pure alcohol. As one of the most penetrating and persistent odors used in perfumery, use of natural musk is limited to the finest perfumes. The art of its application lies in fortifying the basic odor so that the bouquet appears to remain unchanged during evaporation. Needless to say, experimentation here is quite costly. Cleanup is difficult, requiring camphor or benzaldehyde in alcoholic solution before washing with soap.

Musk primarily imparts lift or life to those blends it graces, rounding out the perfume without dominating. It blends well in oriental or heavy perfumes, alchydic bases, lily of the valley, rose, clover, and violet.

Natural musk is generally used as a tincture in perfume. Musk tinctures are prepared in mechanically stirred containers from 2% to 6% musk grains in 90% alcohol, with the addition of ammonia, lactic acid, animal black or bone black (black pigment made by calcining finely ground animal bones), sugar, and lactose. Maceration goes on for 6 months.

Synthetics include the nitro-musk ambrette, musk ketone, musk xylol, and musk tibetine. The macrocyclic musks, including muscone, are represented by cyclopentadecanolide (Exaltolide), cyclohexadecenolide (Ambrettolide), cyclopentadecanone, oxahexadecanlides, and ethylene brassylate. Musk Xylene was patented in 1888.

The indane group of musk odorants include the tetralin musks such as Givaudan's Versalide and Polak's Frutal Works' Tonalid. Exaltolide (Firmenich), Moskene (Givaudan), Phantolide (P.F.W.), Celestolide and Galaxolide (I.F.F.), Musk R-1 (Naarden), and Oxalide (Takasago) are all excellent. Volume 2 of Arctander's *Perfume and Flavor Chemicals* lists over 80 synthetic musks in Table 3. Musk ketone has the softest odor and widest application in fine perfumes.

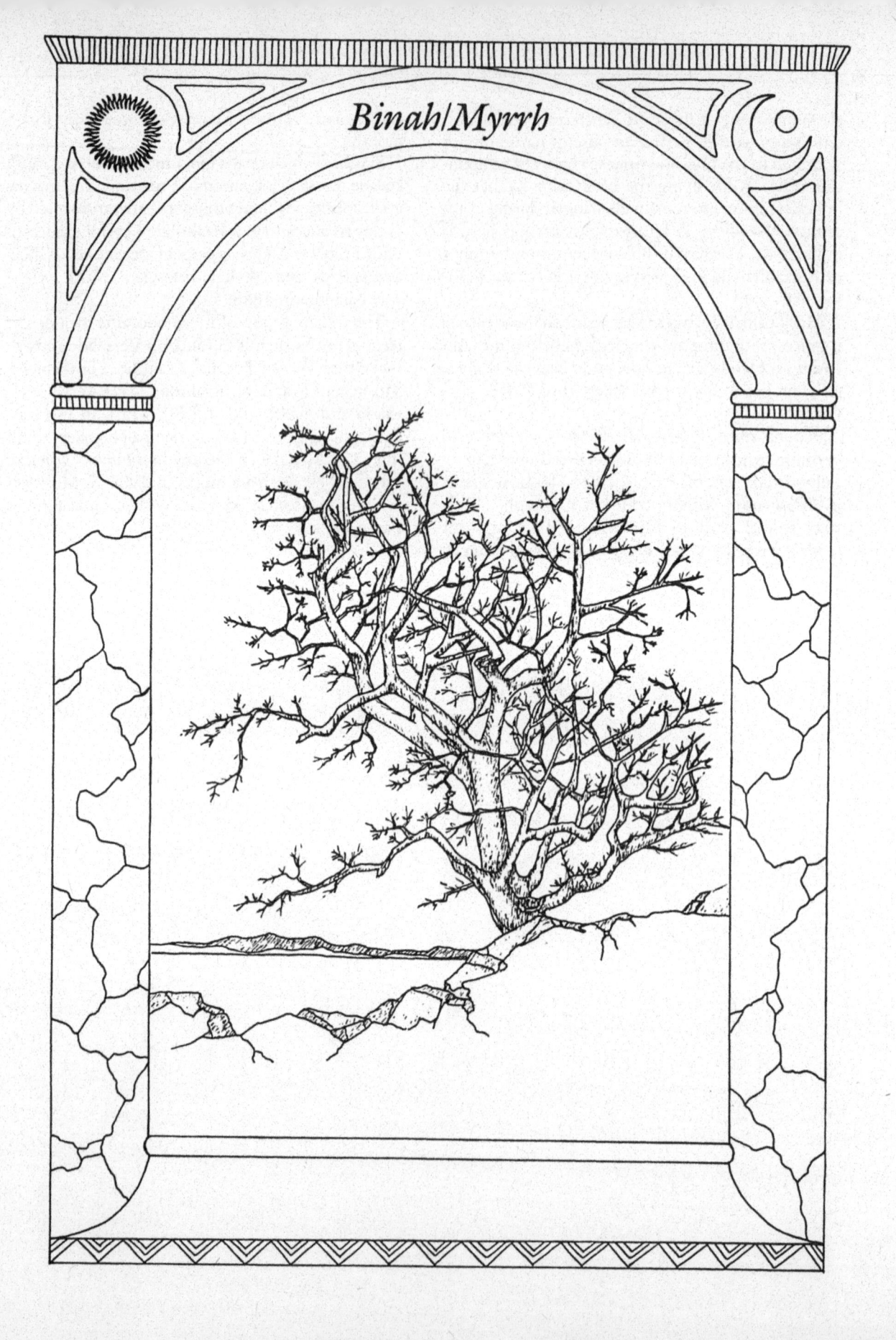

Binah/Myrrh

I will cause to be brought to thee fine oils and choice perfumes, and the incense of the temples, whereby every god is gladdened. Of myrrh hast thou not much; all that thou hast is but common incense. Ashipu came and delivered me, and he gave me a shipload of myrrh, fine oil, divers perfumes, eye paint, and the tails of giraffes.

—Egyptian Papyrus (2000 B.C.) Hermitage Museum, Leningrad

3. BINAH = MYRRH, CIVET

QABALA

Binah represents pure Understanding. It is the divine feminine component of godhead. As such, it is the *yin* basis of all material manifestation, or the principle of form. In terms of human evolution and mysticism, Binah symbolizes the mystical experience of the pure soul finally freed from its entanglement with mind. Detachment from identification with Universal Mind allows the aspirant to "cross the Abyss," or untie the knot between the soul and the mind. This abyss is the gulf between spheres 1 to 3 and 4 to 10 on the Tree of Life, between the purely physical and the most subtle physical manifestation. (see Regardie's *The Middle Pillar*.)

Binah is the true Self, the liberated soul. Also known as Shakti, Shekinah, Maya, Isis, Anima Mundi, or the Madonna, Binah is the energy of the Comforter. Characteristics stimulated by the scents corresponding to this sphere reflect the characteristics of its ruling planet, Saturn. They include understanding, stability, and fertility. A secondary qabalistic attribute for this sphere is the scent of the madonna lily. Juno (Hera) is the goddess associated with Binah. The lily was held sacred to her of whom it was said, "from the milk of her breasts sprang this beautiful flower." The sorrow of Binah is that the soul is so near, yet so far from Kether and God-realization.

MYRRH

Myrrh is traditionally the odor of sorrow and bitterness; it is the dark and passive side of Binah.

—Aleister Crowley, *777*

DESCRIPTION

Myrrh is an exudate that forms naturally in various small trees and shrubs of the Commiphora species (*Burseraceae*). The yield is increased by incisions made in the bark. It is the most ancient gum resin known. It is sometimes used as a straightforward tincture but is also available as a resinoid, oil, and absolute. Among its constituents are cuminic and cinnamic aldehydes; esters of formic, acetic, and other acids; eugenol and metacreosol; limonene, dopentene, pinene; and probably two or more sequiterpenes. Do not confuse it with the so-called Bisabol myrrh, which is now called opopanax.

Myrrh trees, found on parched rocky hills, grow 4 to 20 feet tall, with a trunk diameter of one foot. The tree bears white to light green flowers in late August or early September. The bark contains numerous resin ducts that are tapped for the myrrh, a yellowish fluid.

Exposed to the air, the resin solidifies into globules called tears. These tears are collected inland in the dry summer months and exported from the coast in winter. Myrrh appears in commerce as yellowish or grayish brown pieces. Myrrh is an oleoresin gum containing 25% to 45% resin, 3% to 8% essential oil, and 40% to 60% gum.

GEOGRAPHIC LOCATION

Somalia, Ethiopia, the Sudan, southern Arabia.

HISTORY

Myrrh is mentioned as far back as 3700 years ago and has a long, colorful history. Its name is derived from the Arabic *murr*, meaning bitter. The myrrh of present-day commerce comes from *C. myrrha* of Somaliland. In former times Arabian myrrh, from *C. nolmol*, was also commercially important. Chosen by the Magi as a gift for the Christ child, myrrh was highly esteemed in the Near East and Mediterranean region. Employed in costly incenses, cosmetics, and perfumes, it was also used in medicines and for embalming.

Myrrh is the first scented plant mentioned in the Bible, where it was called bdellium. The Greeks called it balsamodendron. Myrrh was valued from earliest times as the only substance available at the time that could provide a powerful and lasting scent. Myrrh originally came from Babylonia, at one time the center of the spice and perfume trade.

When the Arabian peninsula came under the dominion of Solomon, the Queen of Sheba made an arduous 2,000 mile journey to secure her trade routes to Egypt, the major market for the aromatics her country grew. She brought seeds of the precious myrrh to Solomon, and these were propagated.

In Egypt's Heliopolis, city of the sun god Ra, incense was burnt three times daily to mark stations in the sun's journey; myrrh was used at high noon. Myrrh is also cited by Democritas as an ingredient in the most famous Egyptian blend, kyphi (or khepri). For mummification, the stomach of the corpse was filled with myrrh and cassia before being sown up.

The Jews learned the sacred lore of fragrances during their captivity in Egypt. Purification rites of Hebrew women accounted for high consumption of aromatics. The purification takes place throughout the year; oil of myrrh is used for half the year, and other aromatics follow. As a bride, Esther underwent this process. In many countries with water shortages where people could not bathe as often as they liked, myrrh was suspended from the neck where body heat caused the fragrance to diffuse. In Arabia myrrh is still collected as it was in Solomon's time: the sticky exudate is combed from the beards of goats who nibble at the shrub.

The Greeks valued myrrh as the main ingredient of a most famous, costly unguent, *megalaion*. An equally prized ointment was called *susinum*, made from red-flowered lilies and myrrh. The Greek ointment, under the name of *susinon*, was still popular in Rome around 450 B.C. The Greeks mixed myrrh infusion in wine in hopes of maintaining sobriety, while the Romans added oil of ben, calamus, honey, cinnamon, and saffron to it.

SCENT AND APPEARANCE

Myrrh has a slightly bitter-astringent, mainly balsamic-resinous character, recalling orange flower and petitgrain. It is a typical oleo-gum-resin containing 3% to 8% essential oil, ⅔ gum, and ⅓ resins. The irregular tears of myrrh are medium yellow to dark or reddish brown color, usually covered with a yellowish dust. Their odor is warm-balsamic, sweet, and somewhat spicy-aromatic; it is also somewhat sharp or pungent when fresh, but never terebinthine (like turpentine). Crude myrrh can be processed into myrrh absolute, myrrh oil, and myrrh resinoid.

MYRRH RESINOID is a very dark, reddish orange-brown viscous mass, hardly pourable at room temperature. Soft and sticky, its odor is intensely warm, deep-spicy, balsamic, aromatic, and very rich.

MYRRH ABSOLUTE is extremely dark reddish brown or orange. A viscous mass, it is slightly more plastic than the resinoid, but still unpourable if free of solvents.

MYRRH OIL is the essential oil steam distilled from crude myrrh. It is pale yellow to pale orange or amber. Not very viscous, it smells warm-spicy with a peculiar sharp-balsamic, slightly medicinal top note. Its sweetness increases to an aromatic, deep, warm-spiciness during dryout, but it is not very tenacious.

BLENDING

Myrrh absolute is prepared by alcohol extraction of resinoid, which is then filtered. So-called myrrh tinctures are not perfume-grade products. Myrrh absolute and concentrated extracts are used in perfumery in the same way as myrrh resinoid. Some suppliers advertise inferior myrrh extracts as myrrh oil. True myrrh oil is steam-distilled and free of contaminants, which cause turbidity in perfume.

Myrrh oil is used in small amounts in perfumes of the heavy floral type, heavy oriental type, and woody-balsamic bases, and it is excellent in high-class forest notes, moss notes modified with cypress oil, juniper oil, and mandarin petitgrain oil. It is occasionally used in oral preparations such as washes.

Myrrh resinoid is processed from the highest-quality crude botanical. Made from true, or heerabol, myrrh, it should be free from odorless foreign matter. The resinoid is extracted with benzene, petroleum ether, or ethyl alcohol. Its intense color is a drawback, as it will darken light perfume blends, yet it is an excellent fixative and sweetener for oriental-spicy bases, chypres, woody bases, forest notes, and pine fragrances. Blend it with cinnamic alcohol, geranium oil, linalool, nitro musks, patchouli oil, spice oils, and the heavier floral perfume bases.

CIVET

DESCRIPTION

Civet is the alternative scent attributed to Binah. We can see myrrh as representing the Dark Sterile Mother and civet as her other aspect, Bright Fertile Mother, because of civet's relation to animal reproduction. Binah, of course, represents Mother Nature in her most exalted sense, as Celestial Queen.

Civet is obtained from the glandular secretion of the civet cat, *Viverra civetta*, and from the horns of bullock, buffalo, or zebu. A soft, pastelike substance, civet has a skatolic odor because of methyl indole or skatole, and it contains a musklike lactone, civettone. Tinctures and anhydrols of civet are used, the infusion being 3% to 6% in 95% alcohol. It is warmed, stirred, and matured for several months.

GEOGRAPHIC LOCATION

Ethiopia, primarily. Civet is obtained from male and female civet cats, preferably the male of the Abyssinian variety. Smaller quantities are collected from other species of civet cat in India, Indonesia, Malaya, China, the Belgian Congo, Somalia, Kenya, and occasionally Haiti.

HISTORY

Annual production of civet is several tons, ranking it among the 20 most important perfume raw materials. Of animal origin, it has been known in Europe since the early part of the sixteenth century, though its origin was at first mysterious. In 1688, a European pharmacist named Pomet sought to confirm the rumor that it came from the civet cat by keeping one for a year. He kept it in a cage, collecting civet from its pouch at his own peril. For this year of hazardous duty he gathered an ounce and a half.

During the sixteenth and seventeenth centuries the Dutch were the main distributors of civet in Europe. The civet was largely imported, but some Amsterdam merchants kept civet cats in cages and collected their secretions. The resulting product was certified as being pure. Still, many people did not know the origin of civet before the report of Lemery, a French chemist of the seventeenth century.

> The beast from whence it is taken is called in Latin, Hyaena, Catus Zibethicus, in English, Civet-Cat. Merchants buy the young ones and breed them tame, so that a cat that is large and gentle may come to be valued at between four and eight pounds sterling.
>
> The best civet is made in England, but great quantity is sent from Holland. The West Indian, Barbadian and African civets are next to goodness, but the blackest is the worst that comes from the East Indies. It is much to be preferred to musk because the scent is finer. It comforts the spirits and is good against all diseases of the head and brain.

One of the earliest uses of civet in Europe was for the perfuming of glove leather. The Italians and Spaniards excelled in this art. By the eighteenth and early nineteenth centuries civet essence was used by many men of fashion. Cowper alluded to the practice in the following lines:

> I cannot talk with civet in the room,
> A fine puss gentleman that's all perfume;
> The sight's enough, no need to smell a beau
> Who thrusts his nose into a raree show.

Highly valued over the years, civet is one of those substances still used in the modern practice of witchcraft, or Wicca. An aphrodisiac recipe for burning in one's bedchamber begins with mixing powdered

Binah/Civet

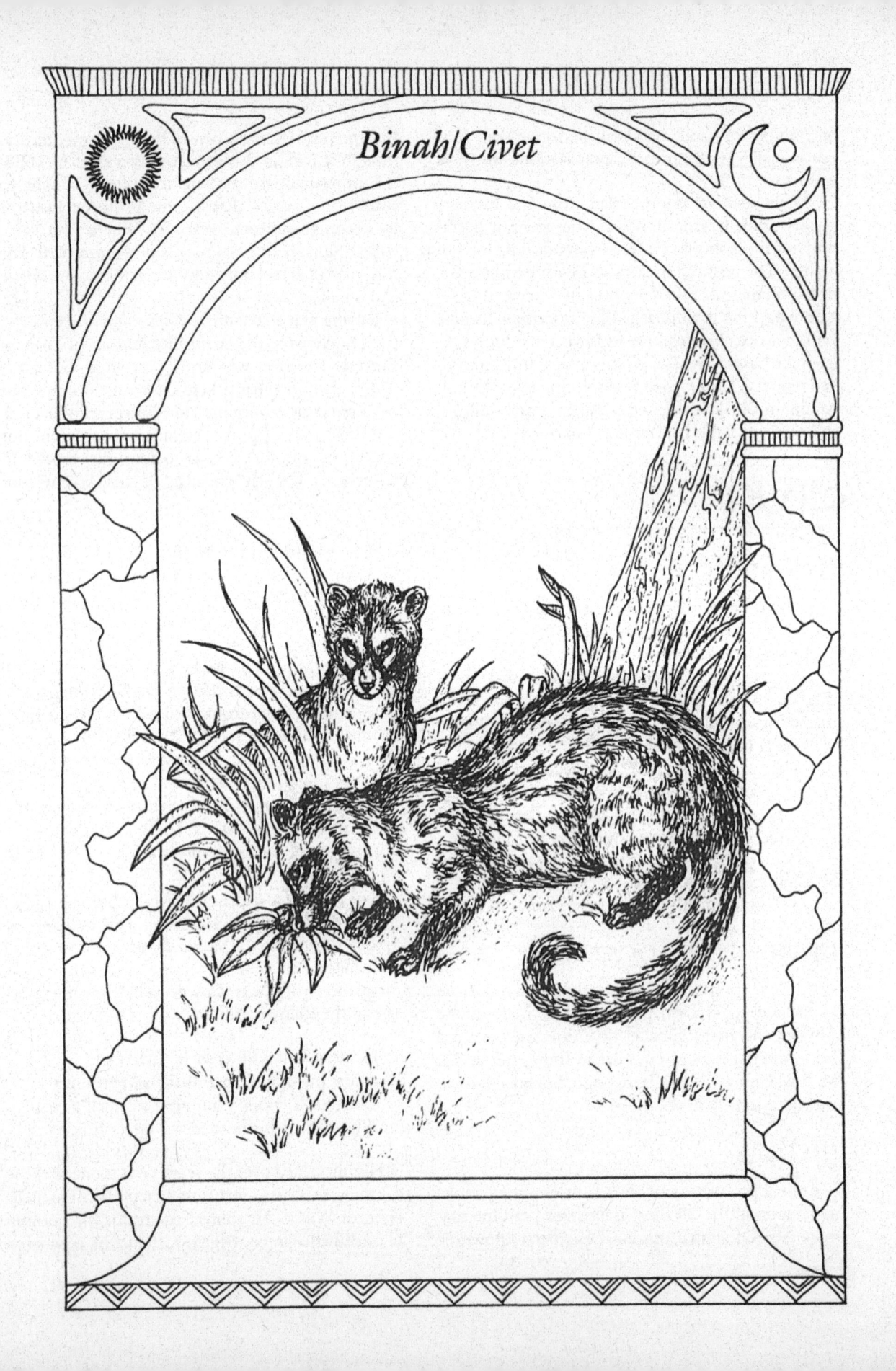

musk, salt, civet, and bits of sandalwood. Then add dried petals of orange blossoms and roses. It is recommended in Sarah Morrison's *The Modern Witch's Spellbook* (pg. 50) that this oil be consecrated before use with the following words:

> O Lord of the Heavens, the Earth
> The great waters of the Sea,
> Sanctify this perfume
> So that anyone who breathes it
> Will be cleansed of evil thoughts and
>   intentions,
> And dream only of love.
> Consecrate the flowers of the scent
> So that a devil who breathes their odors
> Can make no mischief,
> This I beseech you,
> Oh Lord of the great Heaven
> And Earth
> And Seas.

In Ethiopia, civet is alleged to have aphrodisiac properties, so a large quantity is consumed locally. Arab women use it cosmetically on their eyebrows and hair.

SCENT AND APPEARANCE

Fresh civet is yellowish white but darkens and hardens as it oxidizes. It has an obnoxious animal odor, but in minute quantities it is pleasant and attractive, and it makes an excellent fixative. The characteristic odor comes from the ketone zibetone. Buyers of crude civet must be alert for adulterations with paraffin jelly and mucilage from gum acacia, honey, beeswax, lanolin, banana pulp, coconut fat, and butter. Civet ready for use appears as a strong (3%) tincture or as civet absolute.

Civet absolute is extracted with a solvent, then purified. It is a black or deep brown viscous liquid with the characteristic odor. Dilute it with alcohol or an odorless solvent to cut its strength to usable proportions. All quality civet products should be typically animal-sweet, with no hint of fecal or urine smells. Though civet is rich and tenacious, collections of natural civet requires cruelty to the cats. For this, and for economic reasons, you may opt to use synthetic civets.

Civettone and Civettol duplicate some of the civet notes but do not fully capture its essence. The warmth, smoothness, and diffusive capacities of natural civet are hard to incorporate, but these are substitutes free of fecal notes. Civet anhydrol is available at uniform quality and cost as a viscous, almost odorless liquid (fixative). There are simple and complex civet formulae, but they all contain at least indole, skatole, tetrahydroparamethyl quinoline, phenylacetic acid, and the ketone civettone.

BLENDING

Concrete of civet is produced from crude product with hydrocarbon extraction. This is further processed with alcohol into civet absolute. Civet tincture is another common form. When using civet, remember its strength tends to grow in a perfume, so add minute amounts and let it mature.

The fixative properties of civet work well in oriental perfumes, honey notes, narcissus bases, and amber types as well as with nitro musks, coumarin, vanillin, and quinoline derivatives. A small amount gives lift and diffusive power to delicate floral bases such as lily of the valley.

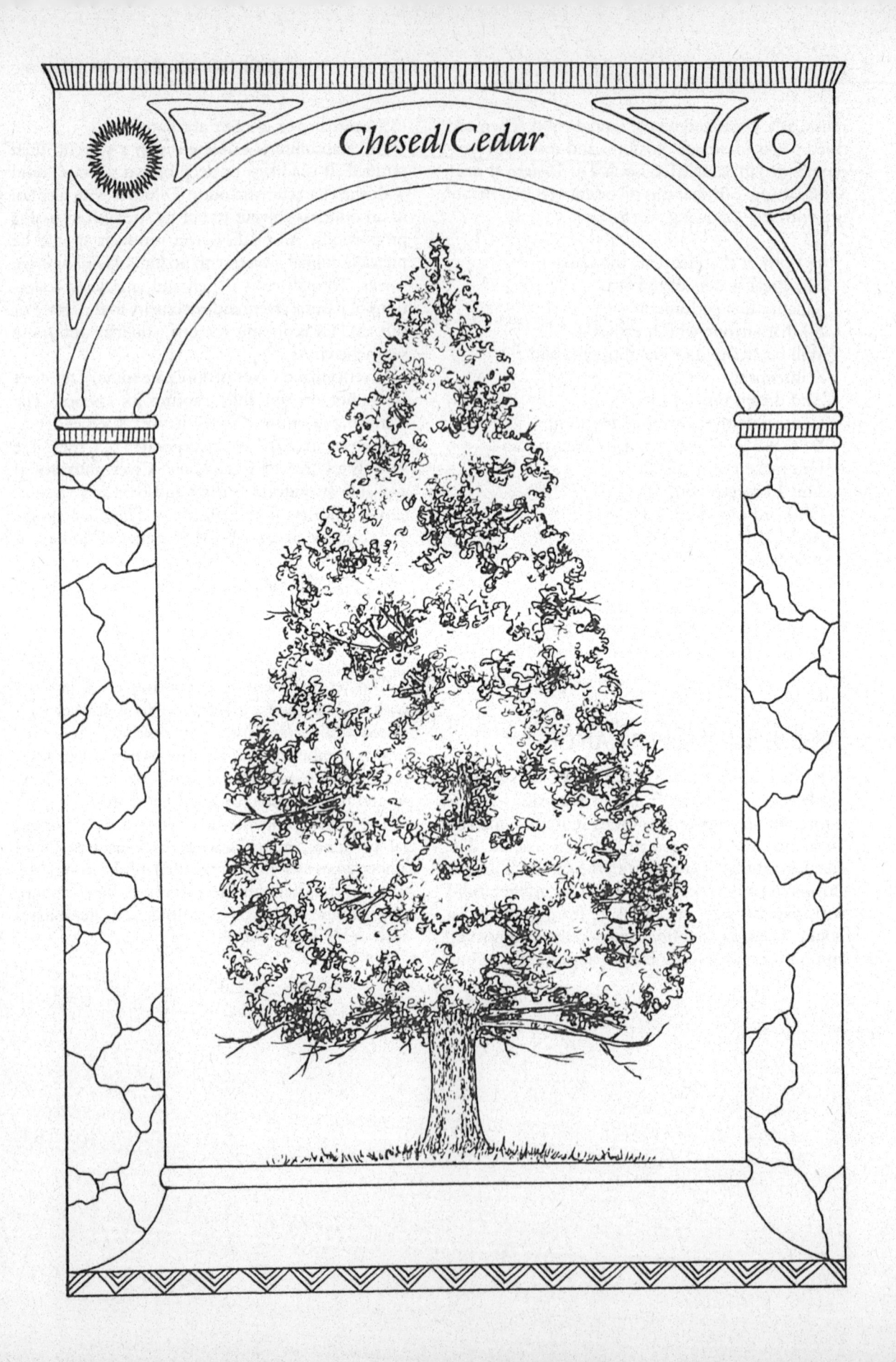

Chesed/Cedar

His countenance is as Lebanon, excellent as the cedars.

—Song of Solomon

4. CHESED = CEDAR

QABALA

Chesed (or Gedulah) is known as Mercy. Ruled by the planet Jupiter and associated with the Greek god Zeus, it is the sphere of the philosopher king. Chesed symbolizes our spiritual and religious needs as well as the tendency toward expansion. Qualities of this sphere include increase, improvement, and growth, both internal and external. It synthesizes insight, knowledge, understanding, and wisdom into the quality of mercy. In mysticism, Chesed is the vision of God-as-king, resplendent on His throne. Keywords include achievement, benevolence, extravagance, healing, justice, leniency, magnanimity, preservation, and respect. Qualities we can stimulate by employing cedar include enthusiasm, good judgment, independence, leadership, nobility, optimism, paternalism, philosophical disposition, self-assurance, wholeness, and wisdom. When you consecrate this essence for magical purposes, remember that Shakespeare wrote, "The quality of mercy is not strained."

DESCRIPTION

The most commonly used cedarwood is *Juniperus virginiana (Cupressaceae)*. There are many other cedarwoods in the juniper, cedar, cypress, and related genera, each with distinctive qualities. One of nature's most handsome creations, cedars grow to great height and spread their branches horizontally for a considerable distance. The evergreen leaves appear in small tufts like those of the larch. Essential oil is produced by steam distillation of the chips and dust of the wood. The main chemical constituent, cedrol, crystallizes in old or cold oil.

GEOGRAPHIC LOCATION

Virginia cedarwood oil is produced in the United States, where it is also distilled. Atlas cedarwood oil comes from Morocco. Still other types originate in Kenya, northern India, Afghanistan, Pakistan, Japan, Oregon, northern California, and Texas.

HISTORY

Cedar was considered an imperishable wood by the ancient Egyptians, who thought it would preserve human bodies enclosed in it. Cedar oil was also injected into corpses during the mummification process. The pharaohs coveted it for making the doors of their temples and building ships. Used frequently for coffins, it is still known by some as coffinwood. The fragrant wood was used as incense in the temples, and the oil was included in the most expensive cosmetics of the Egyptians.

In 2700 B.C. a pharaoh sent 40 ships to Tyre to import cedar trunks. The tree was so important that Cheops I sent an expeditionary force to Canaan in 2350 B.C. to prevent a Bedouin attack that might disrupt trade routes. By 1950 B.C. Sesotris I ensured the supply lines by subjugating Canaan and the port of Tyre.

Solomon's temple was made exclusively of cedarwood stripped from the forest of Lebanon. Harvesting by the Egyptians and the Jews decimated the Lebanese forest, which has never recovered. The last trees are believed to have been used for the Temple of Diana at Ephesus. This wonder of the ancient world burned wildly on the night of the birth of Alexander the Great.

Horace speaks of books being preserved with cedarwood oil and of keeping books in cedar chests. The ancients had a proverb that great writing was "worthy of being cased in cedar." Herodotus recorded the cosmetic use of cedar by Assyrian women. They ground the wood with cypress and frankincense, mixed in a little water, and anointed themselves with this sweet-smelling, skin-softening paste.

In more recent times production of cedarwood oil has increased in the United States. Oil production from northern California and Oregon stands of Port Orford Cedar peaked between the world wars. Lately most of this cedarwood has been exported to Japan, where it is sunk in harbors to preserve it for future use.

SCENT AND APPEARANCE

The varieties of cedar are so different that they must be dealt with separately.

CEDARWOOD ATLAS RESINOID and Atlas cedarwood oil (Moroccan cedarwood oil) come from *Cedrus Atlantica*. The resinoid is a highly viscous, dark amber to brownish fixative. The absolute is a very viscous liquid that is brownish yellow. They both carry some solvent odor but are not camphoraceous and do not have the sharp ketone top note found in the essential oil. The oil is yellowish to orange yellow or deep amber, viscous, and sometimes turbid. The odor is overpowering when undiluted, having a very woody camphoraceous smell. There is a sweet and tenacious woody undertone that lacks the delicateness or depth of florals.

EAST AFRICAN CEDARWOOD OIL, from Kenya, is very dry-woody, somewhat earthy, with a strong top note. It is the "lead pencil" odor. It is less balsamic than Virginia oil, similar to Texas oil.

TEXAS CEDARWOOD OIL, from *Juniperus mexicana*, is distilled from heartwood. Oil comes both crude and rectified. It smells pleasant, sweet-woody, though somewhat smoky or tarlike. It dries with a tenacious sweet balsamic odor with a uniform dryout.

VIRGINIA CEDARWOOD OIL, from the southern red cedar, is a shrub or tree that occasionally grows to considerable size. Sawdust is distilled to an oil that is yellow or slightly yellow-orange. Rectified oil is water white, smelling oily-woody with the sweet balsamic odor of cedar lumber. Virginia oil smells like cedar chests, while Texas oil is sweeter.

HIMALAYAN CEDARWOOD OIL, from *Cedrus deodara*, resembles Atlas oil, with a curious animal note. Japanese oils (hiba, honoki, and sugi oils) are from the genus *Cupressaceae*. Port Orford cedarwood oil is no longer in production. Cedar leaf oil, from *Thuja occidentalis*, is known as thuja oil and has a scent suggesting wormwood, basil, and sage.

BLENDING

The cedarwood oils are extensively used in perfumery. Their mild, woody, and slightly balsamic odor blends well with sandalwood, vetiver, and patchouli and forms the basis of many household and industrial scents. Cedrol and its acetates provide a mild woody-methyl ionone odor.

ATLAS RESINOID AND ABSOLUTE are used with bois de rose oil, boronia absolute, calamus oil, cassie absolute, cistus oil, mimosa absolute or concrete, olibanum, clary sage, vetiver, and ylang-ylang. The Atlas products blend with labdanum for woody, woody-oriental, woody-floral, and violet bases.

EAST AFRICAN OIL is a good fixative for soaps, pine fragrances, and other woody notes. It blends well with rose notes, oriental bases, and moss notes. Use for violet, fougere, and chypre bases as well as woody-aldehydic blends and for modifying vetiver, patchouli, and sandalwood.

TEXAS CEDARWOOD OIL is the preferred oil in America. It is a versatile blender for ionones (violet), methylionones, cinnamic alcohol, nitromusks, amber and leather bases, pine, patchouli, spruce, and vetiver oil. A blend combining cedar

(Chesed) and leather (Geburah) would represent the Causal Plane, perhaps with some added frankincense.

VIRGINIA CEDARWOOD OIL is available rectified and in fractions. The lightest fractions have a very dry top note, while the heavier ones preserve the balsamic-woody odor of cedrenol, another chemical constituent of cedar oil. It is a fixative and cost-reducer for vetiver oil, sandalwood oil, patchouli oil, and guaiacwood oil.

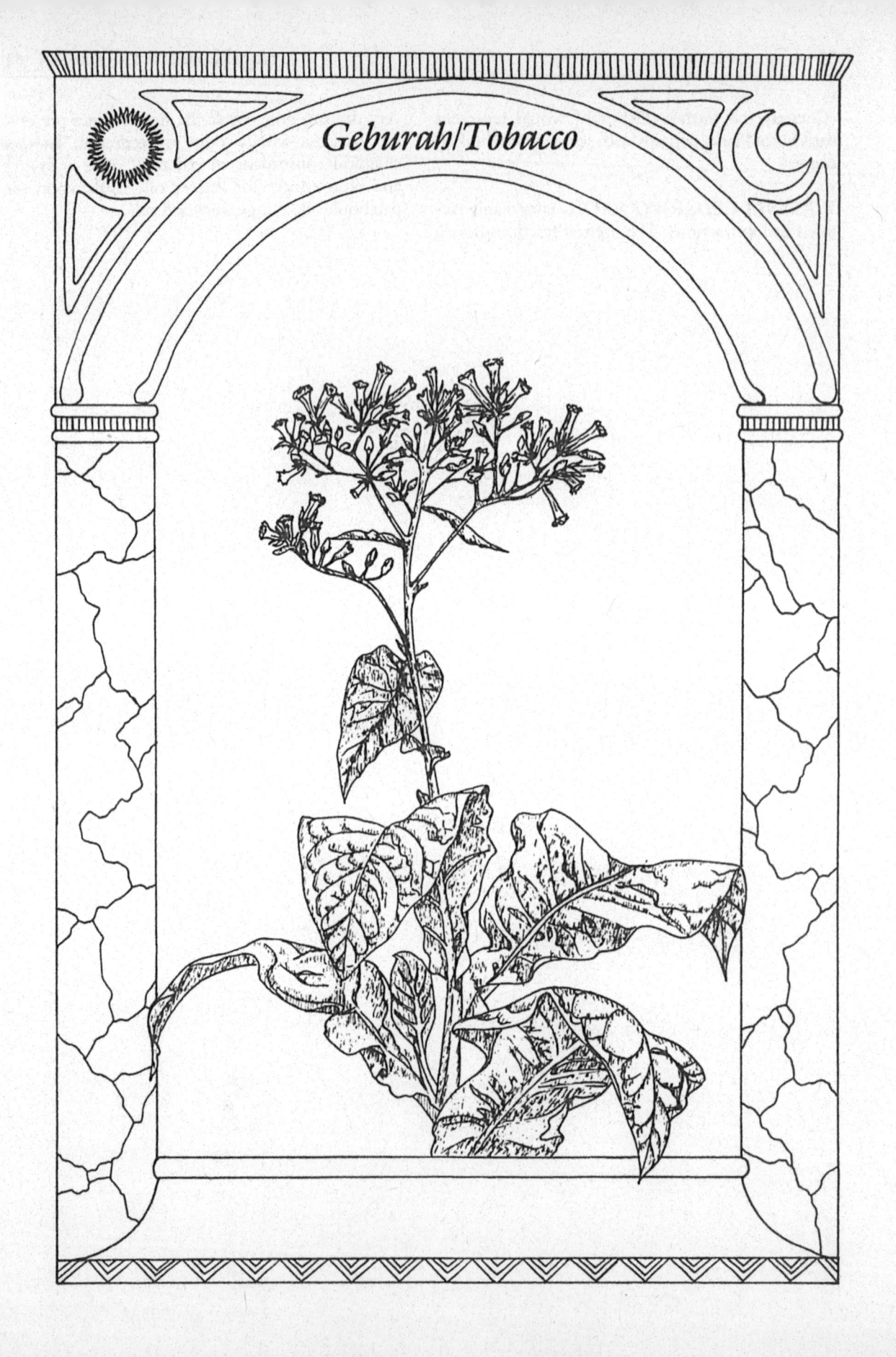

Geburah/Tobacco

"Perfume is a weapon."

—Anonymous master perfumer

5. GEBURAH = TOBACCO, LEATHER

QABALA

The scents of this sphere, which is known as Justice or Severity, reflect the rough-and-tumble life of the Mars-ruled type. Its archetype is the Warrior king and includes soldiers, adventurers, athletes, and others who embody the spirit of the warrior. The militant or warrior type yearns for victory (Netzach) much as Ares yearned for Aphrodite. The spiritual aspects taught in martial arts capture the essence of the sphere Geburah.

The mystical experience of this sphere is brutal self-assessment of your personality from the perspective of your higher Self. Positive qualities of this station to integrate include assertiveness, bravery, courage, devotion to duty, discipline, fitness, fortitude, machismo, obedience to higher authority, power, self-control, self-defense, self-sacrifice, strength, virility, and vitality. Those strong in these qualities are competitive, usually muscular and fit, and have an interest in weaponry and defensive or offensive strategies.

TOBACCO

DESCRIPTION

Nicotiana tabacum, or tobacco flower, is a plant whose perfume is most pronounced in the evening. Tobacco leaf absolute come from *Nicotiana*; it recalls the smell of a cigar and bears some resemblance to the body note of musk. Decolorized absolutes are available.

GEOGRAPHIC LOCATION

This annual plant of the nightshade family originated in North America but is now grown in many places worldwide.

HISTORY

Europeans had their first exposure to tobacco when they saw the Indians of North America using it as a ceremonial smoke. Sir Walter Raleigh brought it back to England, where it promptly gained interest and wide use as smoke and snuff. The use of snuff became very popular in pre-Revolutionary France.

Tobacco also was used widely as a disinfectant and as a preventive of infection. Even children were made to smoke in the belief that this would help them escape the plague. Today, chewing tobaccos are popular; these often have rum and extract of licorice added to improve their flavor.

SCENT AND APPEARANCE

Tobacco leaf absolute is processed from concrete with solvents, mostly in France and the United States. Virginia type leaves are preferred, but Turkish and Syrian are acceptable (latakia absolute). Absolute from concrete is semisolid and dark brown and has a strong, repulsive cigar odor. Distilling yields a paler, amber-colored, viscous liquid. In dilution it has the characteristic tobacco scent.

Anhydrol Tobacco (Givaudan) is a product of this type, though it is somewhat dilute. Resinoine

Incolore Tabae (P. Robertet & Cie.) is another powerful concentrate of this type. Phenylacetic acid is a major component of these products and is used in artificial tobacco flavors.

BLENDING

Tobacco flower is simulated by a variation on the jasmine theme, adding lily components such as lilial, lyral, or cyclamen aldehyde, with small amounts of p. cresol methyl ether or p. cresyl acetate. Absolute of tobacco flowers is unavailable to the public because it is made by a few perfume houses for their own use.

This absolute or its substitutes are used not only in the tabac type of modern or aldehydic perfumes but also for dry or masculine effects in fantasy blends or oriental blends. These materials blend well with sandalwood, castoreum, labdanum, clary sage, vetiver, bergamot, methyl-ionones, and cedarwood derivatives. They produce effects that are very hard to imitate or match with other materials.

LEATHER

DESCRIPTION

Leather or *cuir* bases have continued to be popular and are widely used in perfumery for a masculine flair. There are English leather, Russian leather, and Spanish leather—all derive their main odor from birch tar oil.

GEOGRAPHIC LOCATION

Synthesized in Europe and the United States.

HISTORY

Queen Elizabeth I loved clothes and perfume and patronized Spanish artisans who created fabulous perfumed leathers. First, they made a mixture of oils of neroli, rose, sandalwood, lavender, and verbena, with a hint of clove and cinnamon and diluted it with a half-pint of spirits, adding 4 ozs. of gum benzoin for fixative. Animal skins were then steeped in the perfume. After drying, the skins were spread with a civet and musk paste. This is the historical basis of the famous Spanish leather.

From the white birch, *Betula alba*, an aromatic oil known as Russian leather is derived. The extraction was rubbed on leather book covers to perfume and preserve them. The Russian government guarded the secret recipe for the extraction for years. The rooms in some European libraries (such as those at Oxford) that contain Russian-bound books are still redolent of fragrance.

Perfumed leather accounts for an interesting aspect of the history of perfume making. The rural city of Grasse, France was known for producing hides of good quality. It then began making perfumed leather, from which it evolved into a center for perfume production. The city's artisans cured their leathers with powdered myrtle, which gave the hides a green hue. By the end of the seventeenth century, Grasse held a rich and powerful monopoly on the trade, keeping their perfumery art a secret. Three years of apprenticeship were required to master the art. By 1789 the exorbitant tax on tanned hides caused a change in fashion to delicate fragrances. This persisted into the eighteenth century, when the French Revolution marked the change from individual craftsmanship to industrial expansion and the deluxe perfume trade.

SCENT AND APPEARANCE

Perfumers often speak of leather notes or leather perfume types. Originally the terms referred to the smell of untanned leather, but they came to mean the odor acquired in tanning—phenols are used for preservatives, and natural tars mask the odors of the process. The characteristic smell comes from the tars. Synthetic leather bases that imitate the English, Russian, and Spanish leathers are available in essential oil form, but they are blends, not true essence.

BLENDING

In France, the leather notes are known as *cuir* or *cuir de russie*, but none of the commercial products are based on natural leather. Birch tar oil fractions, castoreum tincture, various phenols, cresols, creosols, cananga oil, storax, and crude amber oil are used in the artificial reproduction of the leather odor type.

Make your own Spanish leather by immersing chamois in the following mixture for ten days.

```
   5 parts rectified birch tar oil
  25 parts sandalwood oil
  20 parts bergamot oil
  20 parts petitgrain oil
  10 parts lavender oil
   5 parts clary sage oil
   4 parts coumarin
  10 parts rose synthetic
 900 parts industrial alcohol
1000
```

Drain and dry the leather on a piece of glass, then spread thickly with the following and press until it dries. This mix can be modified with patchouli, labdanum, oakmoss, jasmine, musk, neroli, or olibanum, among other scents.

```
 150 parts amber liquid
  50 parts olibanum r.
 200 parts glycerine
 350 parts rose water
 250 parts acacia powder
1000
```

Formula from Poucher and Howard, *Perfumes, Cosmetics, and Soaps*, pp. 296–297.

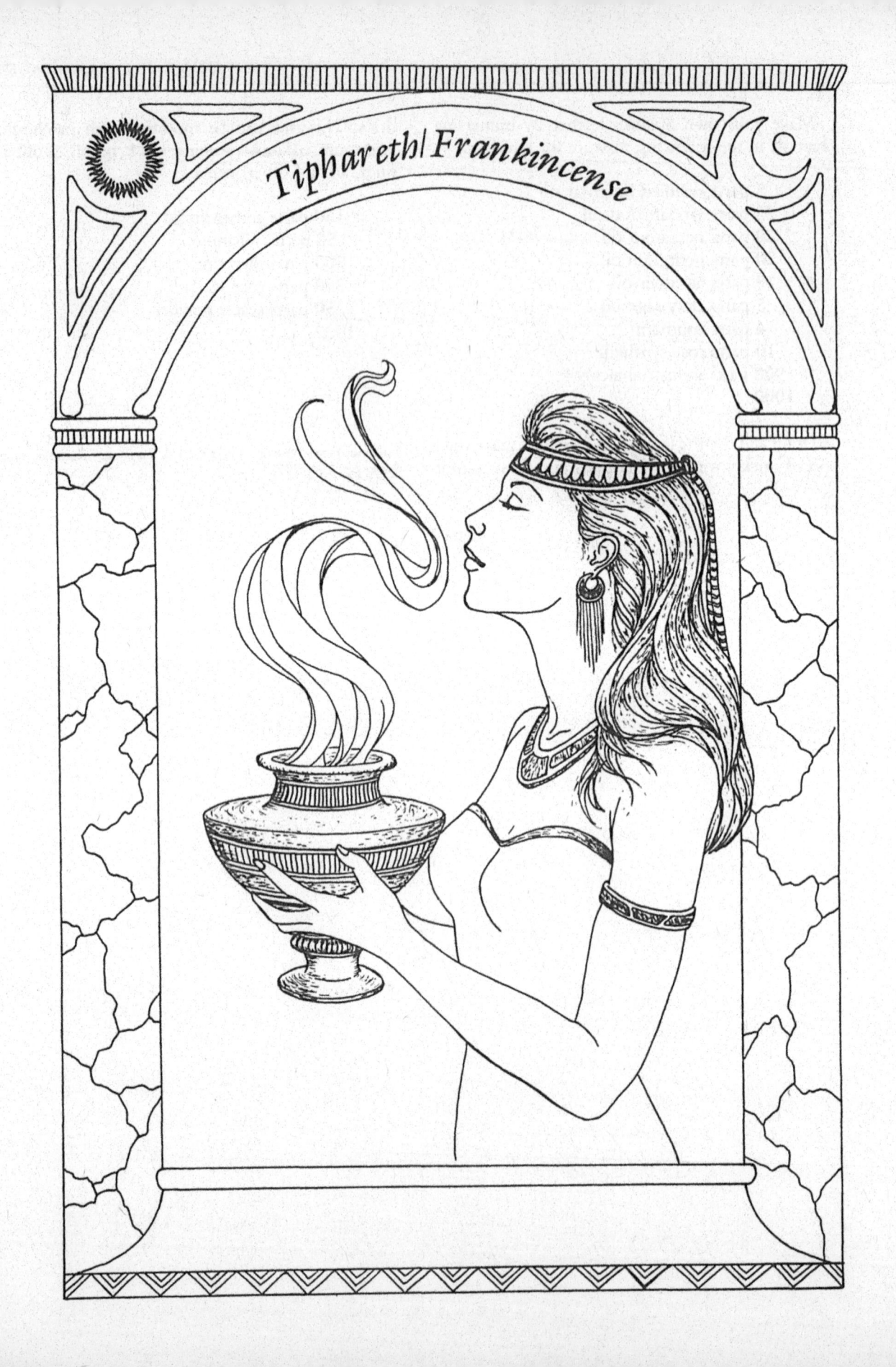

Tiphareth/Frankincense

The Magi came from the East, bringing gold, frankincense *and* myrrh.

—The Bible

6. TIPHARETH = OLIBANUM

QABALA

Tiphareth, Beauty, represents the integrating principle of the higher Self. Associated with the sun, it is the light of higher consciousness. In the mystical experience of Tiphareth you encounter your own higher self and sacrifice your personal desires. You realize the greater Reality and begin to integrate it into your daily life. Initiation into Tiphareth implies a period of trial and purification during which you learn to stabilize contact with the Self. It means transformation of personality. The animal nature is sublimated to the spiritual drive, therefore Tiphareth is associated with self-realization.

Other correspondences include solar deities such as Apollo, Christ, Mithras, Krishna, Osiris, and Buddha. The qualities of Tiphareth are balance, beauty, bliss, creativity, devotion, enlightenment, freedom, harmony, healing, inner guidance, integration, intuition, joy, meditation, radiance, realization, rebirth, reflection, redemption, sanctification, sexual and spiritual ecstasy, transcendence, transformation, truth, volition, and wholeness. The solar quality of this sphere is reflected in the glorious odor of the original temple incense, frankincense (olibanum), still used in the Catholic church.

DESCRIPTION

Frankincense is an aromatic gum resin obtained from trees of the genus *Boswellia*, family Burseraceae, found in the Middle East, Africa, and India. To harvest the frankincense a deep incision is made in the trunk of the tree, and a five-inch piece of bark is peeled off. Milky juice exudes and dries in the air, then the incision is deepened. As the resin sets up, it is gathered from May through September. The largest globules are of the best quality and are kept separate from the resin that runs down the tree. The Arabian resin harvest is exported from Arabian ports, shipped to Bombay, then to Europe, China, and other parts of the world.

Frankincense is sold as semiopaque, oblong tears or irregular lumps covered with white dust. The pieces have an amorphous internal structure with color ranging from dull yellowish brown to a purer, green-tinged, almost colorless look. Larger lumps have more surface area, therefore their essential oils have more chance to volatize. Dust and siftings yield little and poor oil. To make essence from crude olibanum requires skill in assessing all grades of frankincense.

GEOGRAPHIC LOCATION

Originally the most desirable olibanum came from southern Arabia. It is also found in western India, Somalia, north-east Africa, and Ethiopia.

HISTORY

Frankincense has one of the longest histories of any fragrance. The ancients valued it as an incense and the demand for it exceeded that for myrrh by five to one. Egyptians employed it in religious ceremonies, but it was not used in the embalming process. Pliny and Avicenna referred to its medicinal uses and the Chinese esteemed it as well, but it has been proven devoid of active medicinal properties.

Carried from Yemen along the Incense Road, frankincense was the second most prized gum of the spice-rich area. Around 1,000 B.C. the Queen of Sheba had to travel the 1,200 mile road along the Red Sea to placate Solomon and protect her trade route.

The Jews adapted the Egyptians' sacramental use of perfumes. It was decreed that only pure frankincense could be used for holy incense. Frankincense constituted one-quarter of the incense of the sanctuary and is frequently mentioned in the Pentateuch. While wandering in the wilderness, the Jews traded other aromatics they had collected for frankincense. It is mentioned 22 times in the Bible.

According to Herodotus, frankincense burned on the altar at the Tower of Babel. Frankincense was widely offered as tribute to both divine and political powers. Frankincense also burned on the Greek altars at Eleutherae in the Temples of Zeus and Demeter. Theophrastus (370–285 B.C.) tells us that frankincense was imported to Greece by the Phoenicians. This trade peaked in Alexander's time, when unguents from Alexandria, Syria, and Pergamus circulated through the empire.

English lore says that Edward the Confessor donated a portion of the frankincense offered to Christ by the Magi as a relic for Westminster Abbey. English sovereigns (and now the Lord Chamberlain) offer up frankincense for the Feast of the Epiphany on January 6. Edward I is recorded as officiating in 1299; an offering of frankincense in 1742 was cited in the *Daily Post*. Even the Reformation church used frankincense, according to Malcolm's *Londinium Redivivum* (1603).

SCENT AND APPEARANCE

The sacred use of this resin never restricted its widespread use in perfumes. Olibanum resinoids, absolutes, and oils are available. Its balsamic odor has a lemony top note with a smooth but pungently fresh and crisp incense note. It is ideal for oriental, woody, powdery, spicy, aldehydic, citrus, and floral perfumes.

OLIBANUM RESINOID is extracted with benzene, which yields a dark-colored product. Results vary depending on whether a hot or cold process is used. This dark amber, orange, or reddish brown extract is plastic but almost solid. It contains all the essential oil of the crude product, about 7% to 10% by weight. Resinoid extracted with petroleum ether is lighter than the benzene extract and makes an excellent fixative. Use at least 4% to 6% in your concoction. It is barely pourable, so the addition of a plasticizer to preserve a liquid state is acceptable.

So-called *olibanum absolute* is made with alcohol extraction. Resin absolute comes from extracting the crude botanical. True absolute is made by extracting the resinoid with ethyl alcohol and processing it further.

Commercially available olibanum absolutes are actually concentrated *tinctures of olibanum* containing unfiltered insoluble matter. This can create problems in mixing; filtered product has superior odor and solubility.

Olibanum absolute is a solid, semiplastic mass of pale amber color with the characteristic frankincense odor. It has no paint-can odor, but a fresh, balsamic, dry and resinous, greenish odor with a fruity green top note and powerful tenacity. Great perfume houses prepare their own absolute as great skill is required.

OLIBANUM OIL, steam-distilled from resin, is pale yellow or pale greenish yellow. With a fresh and diffusive top note, its middle note is green and woody with a hint of turpentine. The mobile liquid is reminiscent of unripe apples. Its pepperiness is mellowed by rich balsamic undertones. The dryout is tenacious, with cistus, amber, and balsamic odors.

BLENDING

OLIBANUM OIL is striking in citrus blends as well as in woody, spicy, and oriental compositions. It goes well in colognes, modifying bergamot and orange. Olibanum and citral make a good base to work from—it is the main base of incense blends and oriental fantasies.

OLIBANUM ANHYDROL and other similar specialties are distilled from olibanum extract. The absolute is a fixative with a lemony special effect; it blends well with cinnamon and other spices. You can achieve a "powder" effect, or powder-like fragrance, by combining olibanum, cinnamon bark, cinnamic alcohol, nitro musks, and coumarin derivatives. Modify with ionones, methylionones, labdanum extract, cistus oil, mimosa absolute, orange flower absolute, or muguet bases. A true oriental note basically includes sandalwood oil, vetiver oil, olibanum absolute, and cinnamon bark. Build on this base with your imagination and style.

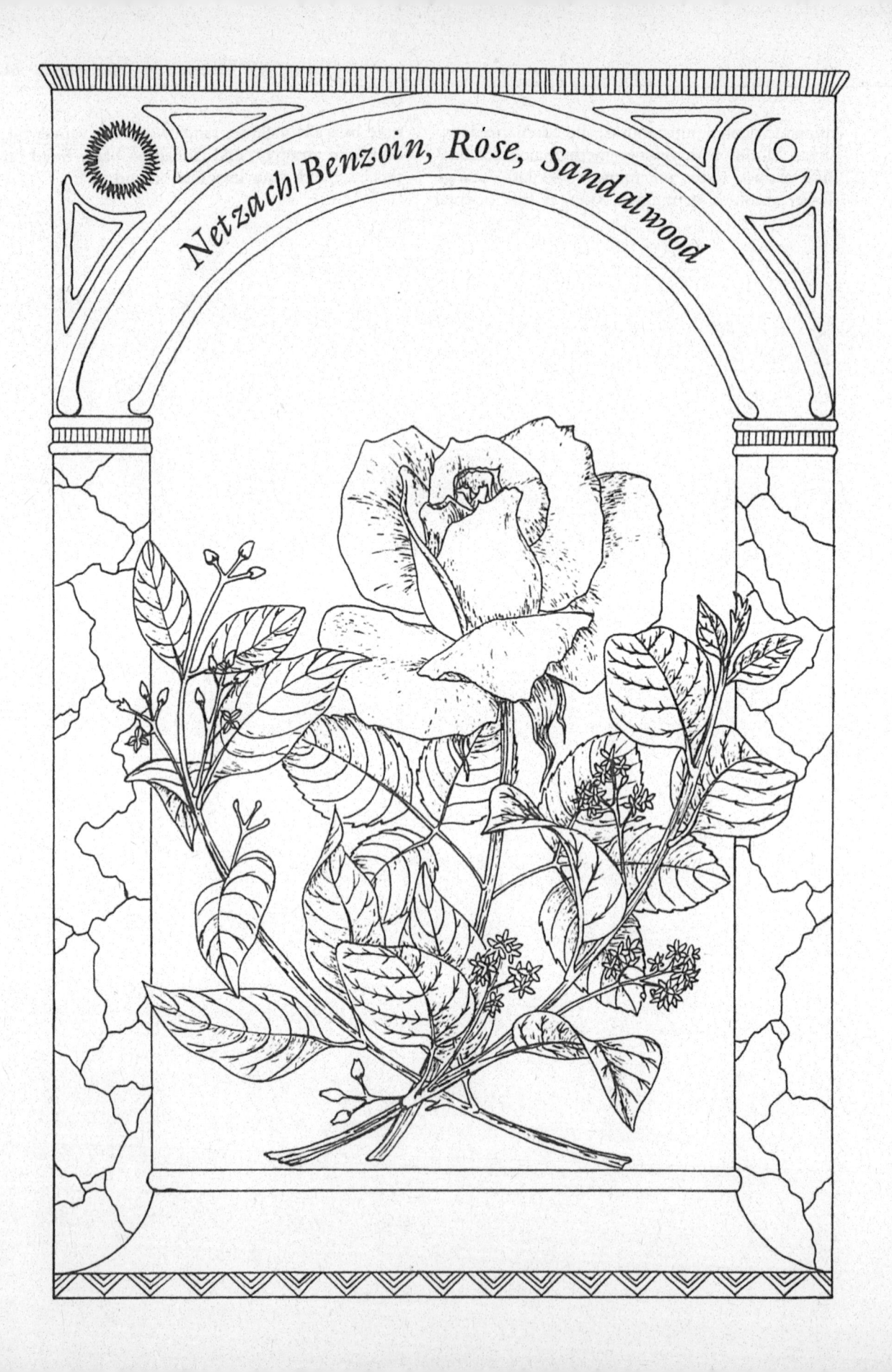

Netzach/Benzoin, Rose, Sandalwood

> *The sensuous seductiveness of* Benzoin *is **unmistakable**... Rose naturally suggests the more physical aspects of the feminine symbol.... Red Sandal is* Venusian, *intuitively by its smell, and sensibly by its color.*
>
> —Aleister Crowley, *777*

7. NETZACH = BENZOIN, ROSE, SANDALWOOD

QABALA

Netzach is usually translated as Victory, but it also means clarity, brightness, sincerity, or truth. The real victory lies through love. Netzach represents the activity of the creative imagination, so this sphere is associated with artistry. Its archetypal image is a beautiful naked Amazon. Venus or Aphrodite, goddess of nature and love, corresponds with Netzach. Qualities or feelings associated with this sphere and stimulated by its scents include achievement, affection, animation, artistry, attraction, beauty, charm, culture, delight, devotion, enchantment, fulfillment, grace, glamor, grandeur, idealism, inspiration, joy, love, nobility, romance, seductiveness, sensuousness, sophistication, soulfulness, style, triumph, and valor.

BENZOIN

DESCRIPTION

Benzoin is a gum resin used to fix and add body to a scent. Trees are tapped when they are six years old or more; each produces about three pounds. Known as benjamin in the perfume trade, benzoin is used as incense in Buddhist and Hindu worship and burned by the wealthy class for pleasure.

Two types of benzoin are Siam benzoin and Sumatra benzoin. Siam benzoin, the best, is obtained as a secretion from an incision in *Styrax tonkinensis*. Its sweet balsamic odor has a characteristic vanilla note. Tears of benzoin range from ivory white to yellow orange or brown. Lower grades are darker and contain debris. Tincture is pale and 95% alcohol soluble. Benzoin resinoids, *clairs*, and absolutes are made by macerating the gum resin in alcohol.

Sumatra benzoin, *Styrax benzoides craib*, has a much greater proportion of cinnamic acid derivatives and coniferyl alcohol. Vanillin is in both varieties. The odor of the Sumatran is coarser than the Siam benzoin, but it has its own applications.

GEOGRAPHIC LOCATION

Siam benzoin is native to Laos and Tonkin; Sumatra benzoin originates in Sumatra.

HISTORY

Benzoin is a main ingredient in one of the most popular perfumes of the modern world, chypre. Based on the rock rose of Cypress, this perfume is fixed with benzoin. Chypre was introduced in Europe by knights returning from the Crusades. Cherished throughout the sixteenth to eighteenth centuries, chypre also contains ambergris, vanilla, Tonka bean, orris, and rose. Chypre recipe for dusting powder includes benzoin, storax, calamint, coriander seed, and calamus root in equal amounts. Musk and civet make modern chypre blends long lasting.

At religious ceremonies, Muslim women burn incense made of benzoin, aloe wood, sandalwood, and patchouli. This, burned at the feet of the dead, is believed to lift the soul to heaven.

Les secrets de Maistre Alexis de Piedmont, the earliest French book on perfume, was published in 1580. Its recipe for damask scent room freshener includes 5 gr. each of musk and ambergris, 2 gr. civet, 4 gr. fine sugar, 1 gr. benzoin, and 3 gr. each storax, calamus, and aloe wood. Powder and cover with damask rose water and simmer slowly.

Elizabeth I carried a pomander of ambergris and benzoin. Benzoin is an ingredient in Spanish leather. Benzoin prevent the rancidity of fats in ointments and pomades. Storax benzoin is the principal source of benzoic acid.

SCENT AND APPEARANCE

BENZOIN TINCTURE is prepared by maceration with alcohol (20 parts tears, 100 parts alcohol). This fixative has a sweet, balsamic vanillin odor. The amber liquid is an antioxidant and is used to heal the skin.

BENZOIN RESINOID can be produced from mixtures of Siam and Sumatra crude botanicals. The extracted and filtered product is hard to evaluate, but this resinoid can be further extracted into alcohol-soluble *Benzoin absolute*. Sumatran benzoins are darker colored, even brown. Resinoid and absolute are frequently adulterated with vanillin, which can discolor certain perfumes.

Siamese product is hard and brittle, almost translucent, and reddish-yellow to pale brown. Selected tears are called tears No. 1; these are the best for perfumery purposes. Sumatran product has several grades, of which almond is best. Being white or cream-colored, the almond shaped tears contain cinnamatest (esters) of coniferyl alcohol, cinnamic alcohol, and benzoresinol rather than the benzoates of the Siam type. Low grades are harsh, like storax. They are dark reddish brown, with little essential oil. Adding a plasticizer to the resinoid is desirable as long as the product is labeled to that effect.

BLENDING

Resinoid is very useful, especially as a fixative for soap perfumes. It can have an odor-depressing effect in some perfumes.

Sumatra is a fixative for fougere (fern), floral-balsamic, and new-mown hay types of scents. It is cheaper than Siam by far, but do not substitute it directly for Siam. Siam is used in delicate scents, whereas the Sumatran type is best in coarser scents such as harsh-balsamic, sharp-floral, and new-mown hay. Siam benzoin is a more effective antioxidant.

ROSE

*'Twas in the bath, a piece of perfumed clay
Came from my loved one's hand to mine, one day.
"Art thou, then, musk or ambergris," I said,
"That by thy scent my soul is ravished?"*

*"Not so," it answered. "Worthless earth was I,
But long I kept the rose's company:
Thus near its perfect fragrance to me came,
Else I'm but the earth, the worthless and the same.*

—Persian poet, Gulistan Sadi

DESCRIPTION

The rose has been called the most perfect of flowers. It is linked to Venus and love. Browning said, "Any nose may ravage with impunity a rose." The Persians cultivated the beautiful red rose; in floral lore the pink rose is that of ardor, or romantic desire. Of the many rose notes, the best include absolute oil of rose de Grasse, Bulgarian rose absolute, Moroccan and Turkish rose absolutes, absolute of rose geranium, and absolute of rose leaves. Rose absolutes are the most widely used of all floral absolutes. The famous Chanel No. 5 is a modern aldehydic perfume combining rose, jasmine, and vetiveryl, among other ingredients. Specialized rose notes include those of the tea rose, Banksiana, Zephyrine, Drouhin, and Marechal Niel types. Red rose is *Rosa gallica* or *rubra*.

Rose petals are harvested at sunrise. While still wet with dew, they are distilled promptly. Seven thousand plants to an acre produce around 5,000 pounds of petals. Five hundred pounds of flowers yield an ounce of attar. Well-tended plants yield for ten years.

GEOGRAPHIC LOCATION

Roses grew in many climes, but the origin of those most used in perfumery are France, Morocco, Turkey, Bulgaria, the Soviet Union, Syria, India, China and the United States.

HISTORY

It is likely that the rose originated in Persia and that Arab nomads spread it throughout the known world. Many anecdotes refer to this cherished flower. It is one of the oldest plants known to mankind yet it has been grown in Bulgaria for only 300 years. In 220 A.D., Athenaeus mentions the strewing of red rose petals eighteen inches deep when Cleopatra first met Mark Antony. Nero spent enormous sums importing dried rose petals for his chambers. When Rome conquered north Africa, cultivation spread to Italy. A hybrid of red rose is painted on the 4,000 year old Palace of Knossos in Crete. The rose, believed introduced to Egypt in the reign of Ramses the Great, has been found in Egyptian tombs. Brought from Syria, it was cultivated by monks for centuries.

Persian gardens were abundant with roses. Persian legend holds that as Mohammed was taken to Heaven, his sweat fell to earth and became the original rose. Damask rose comes from Damascus; Syria means "land of roses."

For the ancient world the rose was a sign of silence. In myth, Eros presented the rose as a gift to the god of silence, and sub rosa, "under the rose," still means keeping a secret. Wealthy Greeks left bequests for the care of their rose gardens. Virgil and Herodotus referred to roses, as did Homer, who mentioned the rose in connection with the apparition of Aphrodite.

Greek interest in perfumes grew when Alexander defeated the Persians and Egyptians around 330 B.C. Apollonius wrote a treatise on the finest perfumes in which he mentioned extract of roses from Cyrene, Phaselis, Naples, and Capua. Pliny told of roses in ointments. Greek physician Marestheus alleged that rose scent would invigorate a tired mind.

Avicenna, an Arabian doctor of the tenth century, discovered distillation and applied his discovery to the rose and other flowers. He created the first attar or otto. Roses were placed with water in a copper alembic and gently heated, distilled, and filtered. In 1187, during the Crusades, Saladin entered Jerusalem, ordering the walls and floor of Omar's mosque to be washed with rose perfume. Bedouin tribesmen still add rose otto to coffee. Arab women use it in eye cosmetics and in an unguent called *urgujja*, which also contains jasmine, sandalwood, and aloe wood.

In Indian mythology, a wife of Vishnu was discovered in a rose. Wealthy Hindu grooms give their brides attar of roses. Abeer (or Abir), a foremost perfume of India used to scent clothes and linens, is made of rose, civet, sandalwood, aloe wood, and zedoary. India's attar is comparable to Bulgarian.

Joan of Arc was given rose petals by the town of Provins in 1429. In the sixteenth century, wide use was made of rose-perfumed pillows, which held orris root, calamus, and a little ambergris, civet, and musk. Henry VIII's perfume recipe is recorded at Oxford: "Take six spoonful of rose oil, the same of rose water and a quarter of an ounce of sugar. Mix well together and add two grains of musk and one ounce of ambergris, then boil slowly for six hours and strain." The Rosy Cross was the famous symbol of the sixteenth century Rosicrucians.

In the nineteenth century, the red rose was used by apothecaries. The House of Lancaster adopted it as the family emblem during the Wars of the Roses (1277). Rose perfume was in great vogue in the Edwardian period. With modern synthetics from geraniol and phenyl ethyl alcohol, there are at least seventeen different rose notes.

SCENT AND APPEARANCE

Rose products include concretes, absolutes, and oils.

DAMASCENA ROSE CONCRETE, from Bulgaria or Turkey, is extracted into a solid, waxy, orange yellow to greenish orange mass that is sweetly floral with a spicyness and a sweet, woody undertone. The deep floral, faintly honeylike note is characteristic. Watch for hard-to-detect adulteration with spent wax, rose de mai concrete, mimosa concrete, or chemicals. *Rosa centifolia concrete* is darkish pale yellow to green or brown-yellow and waxy (melting point 45° to 52°C). Less honeylike than damask, it has a warm, deep floral, slightly woody-sweet scent. Mainly processed into absolute or used in solid wax perfumes.

BULGARIAN ROSE ABSOLUTE is often processed in France. It differs from Moroccan, yielding an orange-yellow to reddish green-yellow viscous liquid. It is warm, spicy, floral, and rosy with honey undertones. A few percent or less in a perfume base is plenty.

MOROCCAN AND TURKISH ROSE ABSOLUTES are half the price of Bulgarian rose otto. A pale yellow or colorless liquid, it smells deep-sweet, with a rich and tenacious floral odor. It isn't as spicy as Bulgarian but has equal warmth. Moroccan oil adds deep warm notes, life, and naturalness to floral and nonfloral perfumes. Watch out for it as a cutting agent in Bulgarian otto.

DAMASCENA OIL, rose otto, or otto of rose is a steam-distilled essential oil. Bulgarian otto is pale yellow to olive-tinged yellow containing crystals of stearopten at temperatures below 21°C. It is warm, deeply floral, slightly spicy, and honeylike. Use 1% in carnation and jasmine bases. You may buy diluted product from middlemen.

ABSOLUTE OIL OF ROSE DE GRASSE (rose absolute, centifolia, rose de mai), from France, is derived from pomade or is extracted with solvents from concrete. The essential oil is further refined. It has a honey note with a delicate peppery note shading off into a natural carnation tone. A hint of green odor depends on the ripeness of the flowers and purity of the crude mass of petals. The concrete is 67% alcohol-soluble absolute. *Rose de mai absolute* is orange to orange-brown-yellow and viscous with a sweet, rich, rosy, tenacious smell. Like Damascena it is honeylike, but it is also less spicy. Diluted, it is delicate, slightly balsamic with a hint of woody undertone that rounds off or lifts dull or harsh synthetic blends.

BLENDING

BULGARIAN ROSE ABSOLUTE is classy and expensive. Used with jasmine, carnation, chypres, orientals, and fantasy bouquets, it makes a superior base. It is so radiant that small amounts add a lot to medium-priced perfumes. Its spent waxes are used in soap perfumery.

ROSE DE MAI ABSOLUTE is used extensively for floral bases, chypres, and orientals, as well as for rounding out synthetics. Use with jasmine, cassia, mimosa, orange flower, and such synthetics as geraniol, citronellol, dimethyl octanol, nerol, phenylethyl alcohol, eugenol, and isobutyl phenylacetate. You can also use it to modify bergamot, clary sage, geranium, sandalwood, guaiac wood, and patchouli.

CENTIFOLIA ABSOLUTE is half the price of Bulgarian and is popular in cosmetics. It can be adulterated with ethyl alcohol. Rhodinol and costus oil, clove bud oil, Peru balsam, and synthetics are common additives. Buy from reputable dealers.

SANDALWOOD

In the Hindu marriage ceremony, the sacred fire is kept constantly burning . . . with sandal-wood, *perfumed oils, and incense, which give off fragrant fumes.*

—C. J. S. Thompson

DESCRIPTION

There are allegedly a red and white sandal, the white being considered more lunar in character, but there is no discussion in the literature of a red sandalwood.* The commercial variety, *Santalum alba*, is the only one available. An east India wood, the best sandalwood comes from Mysore. Oil is steam-distilled from cultivated trees over thirty years old. The trees are parasitic—they attach themselves to the roots of other trees and grow to more than forty feet.

---

*Arctander (1960) describes the so-called red sandalwood as *Pterocarpus santalinus* of India. Since the wood is not fragrant, it yields no essential oil and is therefore not used in perfumery. It has been used as a red food coloring.

GEOGRAPHIC LOCATION

The tree originated in India (Madras and Mysore), Sri Lanka, Indonesia, and surrounding islands; it grows wild in Timor and Celebes. Australian sandalwood oil comes from *Eucaria spicata*.

HISTORY

This tree has been cultivated in India for thousands of years. It is mentioned in the oldest Vedic works from the fifth century B.C. Its oil was used to embalm princes of Ceylon in the ninth century. In solid form, the odor lasts for years, making it a valuable trade good. Used in India to build temple gates, it is immune to the attack of white ants. The gate at Somnath dates from A.D. 100 and still stands today. Sandalwood is used in the rituals of Vishnu and for cosmetics.

Sandalwood, or santal-wood, blends well with rose and so was used to adulterate attar. As a spirit, it is used for orientals—heavy perfumes with an eastern quality. The once dense sandalwood forests of India, Burma, and China were used up, and it now has to be imported from Indonesia. It is a favorite incense and is used ceremonially with rose otto to wash away sins on the last day of the Hindu year (April 12). It purifies body and soul.

Chips collected during the felling of trees yield about 30 ounces of otto for every 100 pounds of wood. Sandalwood shavings are allowed to lend their scent to many kinds of flower petals awaiting distillation. The scented talcum powder Abeer is a favorite of Indian households.

In Moslem countries, sandalwood and other ingredients are placed in a censer at the foot of the dead to carry their soul heavenward. Sandalwood ointment is rubbed on the dead, and the wealthy burn it on their pyres. The poor must use juniper.

An Indian folktale tells of a poor blind man who chopped firewood to sell. In return for an unselfish kindness, a nobleman rewarded him with a grove of these costly trees. He thought this would make him wealthy for life. Imagine the nobleman's chagrin upon his return years later, when he found the blind man had sold the precious wood as kindling for his normal price. This is an allegory of the blessings we receive from God: many times they are blindly squandered.

In Tantric philosophy sandalwood is recommended for men only. The Japanese burn sandalwood and junko wood on the shrines of Buddha and in Shinto religious occasions. Europeans used sandal in Spanish leather. Nineteenth-century scientists discovered the bacteriological property of this oil, it kills bacteria in less than an hour. This oil has a 4,000 year old history of continual use. Known in Ceylon only 1,000 years, it has only appeared in European and American perfumery since the 19th century.

SCENT AND APPEARANCE

This aromatic wood is very sweet, smooth, almost rosaceous, with a uniform dryout. An excellent fixative, it is powerfully tenacious. Australian oil, the source of santalol, is a substitute lacking the soft-sweet top note of Indian. Indian oil is pale yellow to yellow, a viscous liquid with an extremely soft, woody, balsamic odor with no particular top note but a uniform redolence.

BLENDING

Mix with rose, violet, tuberose, clove, lavender, and bergamot as a fixative in woody-floral, oriental-floral, chypre, fougere, clover, carnation, origan, and other bases. It is used to co-distill rose and other delicate flowers. All Indian attars contain sandalwood oil.

Sandalwood makes a background note and fixative for amber perfume and opoponax or precious wood types. Also try with ionones, oakmoss, labdanum, patchouli, vetiver, musks, geranium oils, mimosa, cassia, costus, clove, eugenol, linalool, geraniol, and cyclamel. Look out for adulteration of Indian oil with Australian oil, cedar oil, amyris oil, or others.

As a flavor material it is of little or no importance, but it was used to flavor Sen-Sen, a sickly sweet oriental licorice candy for masking bad breath.

Hod/Liquid Amber

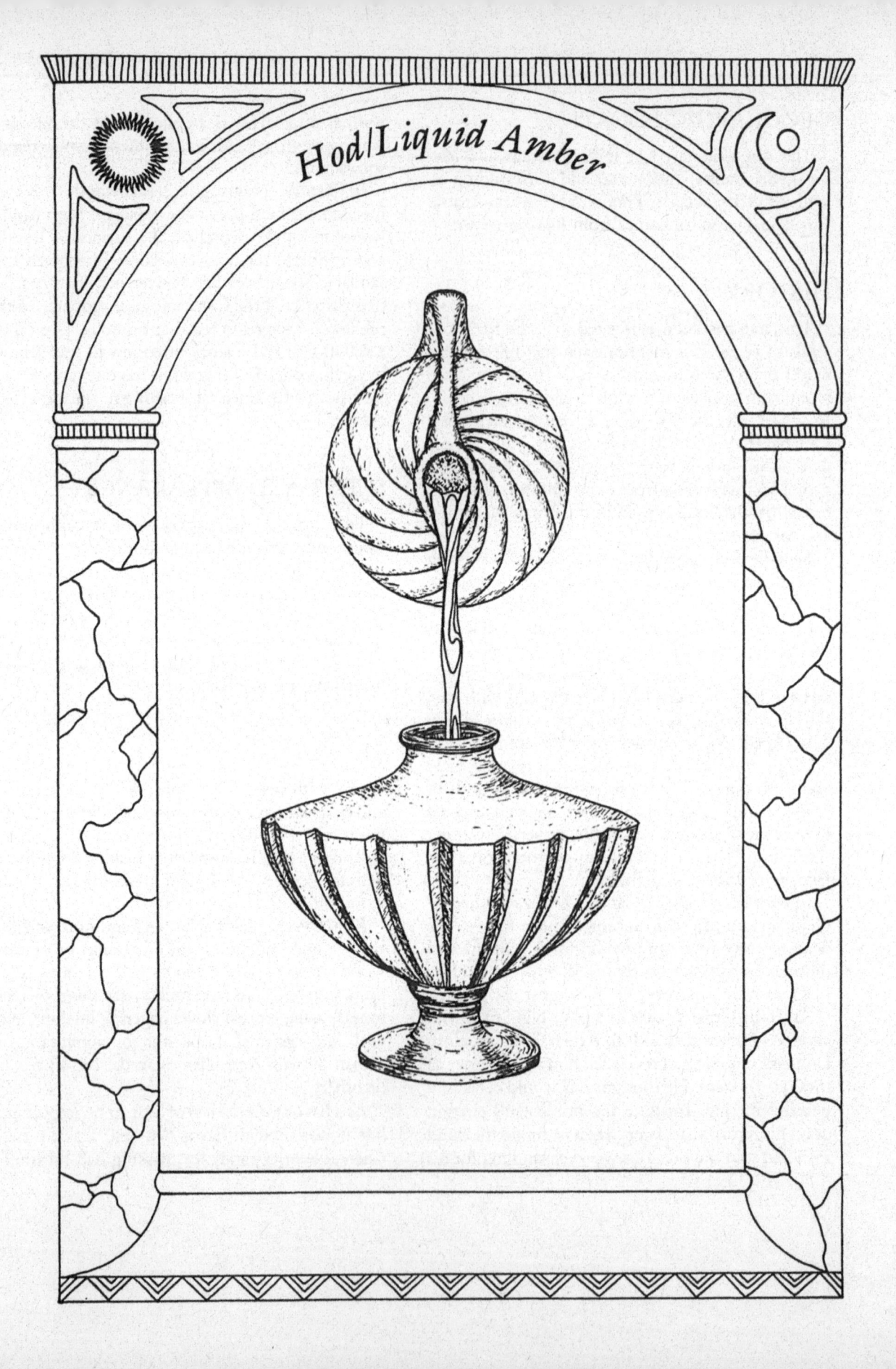

> *Storax is chiefly Mercurial on account of its nondescript nature . . . a menstruum for other perfumes in the same way as Mercury is the basis of amalgams. But storax is really too dark and heavy to be a really adequate perfume for Hod.*
>
> —Aleister Crowley, 777

8. HOD = STORAX

QABALA

Hod is known as Glory. It also signifies renown, praise, honor, or splendor. This sphere of the rational intellect, or mental body, lets you test your theoretical knowledge of the universe experimentally. You learn the power of concentration when working on this station. This is the beginning of identifying with the Self, rather than the personality. The thinking process relies heavily on mental images, so visualization is a keyword. Other qualities and attributes include adaptability, ambition, analysis, communication, dexterity, discrimination, genius, good luck, humanism, humor, initiative, interchange, interpretation, inventiveness, morale, observational ability, opportunism, order, relatedness, skill, synchronicity, will, wit, and writing ability. Other scents for Hod include amber or spikenard, an ancient scent which the magical order of the Golden Dawn and Crowley seemed to ignore in their attributions.*

DESCRIPTION

Storax, or styrax, also known as liquidamber, is a gum resin exudation of *Liquidambar orientalis* (Hamamedlidaceae or witch hazel family). There is also an American variety called *Liquidambar styraciflua*. Both Asian and American types are purified and preheated before use.

Storax is commercially available as resinoid, absolute, and oil. Its chemical makeup includes styrene, benzyl, cinnamyl, and phenylpropyl alcohols with a variety of cinnamic esters, most notably 5% to 10% styracine. Products have a pleasant balsamic odor but the top note smells of benzene due to the styrene. The basic note is almost animal.

The medium-sized storax tree is widespread in Asia Minor. To harvest the storax, the tree is not felled, but bark is removed, then incisions are made in the sapwood. The sap is collected in a can and the peeled bark is boiled to extract more storax. All product is filtered. Packed in cans, the sap is still 25% water, which floats on the top. A sediment sinks to the bottom. In further cleaning, it is extracted with benzene for a true resinoid. Alcohol extraction produces the resin absolute. Extraction with odorless solvent gives a clear, pourable 50% storax resinoid that is soluble in all perfumery materials.

GEOGRAPHIC LOCATION

The tree is native to Anatolia and Asia Minor. There is also an American variety, growing wild in the eastern and southern United States, Mexico, Honduras, and Guatemala. In the latter two countries it is collected for export.

HISTORY

One of the most valued of ancient perfumes, *Styrax officinalis* was burned as altar incense. Storax was

---

*The alternative, spikenard, derived from *Nardostachy jatamansi* of the valerian family comes from Bhutan and Nepal. Traders brought it to Palestine in unguent form, prior to the Christian era. Used only on special occasions, it was valued by all but especially by the wealthy. Produced only in India and Japan, it is in scarce supply and is frequently mislabeled or adulterated.

an ingredient of chypre, a scent widely used in the court of Henry IV of France. It is also recommended for scenting an apartment in the first perfume book by Master Alexis. During the reign of Louis XIII it was used to fumigate bedchambers, being dispensed as a powder from bellows. One recipe for this substance appeared in the anonymous work, *The Charitable Physician* (1629):

½ lb. iris root [orris]; 4 oz. roses; 1 oz. each cyprus root, marjoram and cloves; 4 oz. each yellow sanders and benjamin [benzoin]; 1 oz. storax. Beat them together into a powder.

A recipe for perfuming Louis XIV's shirts was known as *aqua angeli*. Described by Dr. Theodor in *Medical Counsels*, it consisted of aloe wood, nutmegs, cloves, storax, and benzoin boiled in rose water four fingers high. Simmered over a flame for twenty-four hours, it was completed with the addition of water of jasmine and orange flowers and a little musk. The king's shirts were then rinsed in the fragrant water. Commercially, the Near Eastern *Storax officinalis* has been replaced by balsam of storax, or gum storax. The tree was first mentioned in print in 1650 by the Spanish botanist Hernandez. Hernandez said the gum was exuded from the bark like "liquid amber." Taking his cue from this, Linnaeus named the genus. The first horticultural planting was in 1681 in the Fulham Palace garden.

In the American variety, *Liquidambar s.*, the balsam is a result of disease in the tree; the sap accumulates in pockets and is tapped for harvest. Balsam is exported in crude form in five-gallon kerosene tins or secondhand fifty-five-gallon drums. This storax has an undesirable gasoline smell from styrene therefore the Asian variety is preferred. After purification the two are nearly identical.

In modern perfumery, one ounce of storax dissolved in a pint of rectified tincture of storax makes a good fixative for florals like jonquil, tuberose, and lily of the valley. Benzoin from *Styrax benzoin* is similar in effect. Storax is resin processed out of the inner bark of the tree. Natives of the Near East usually collect it and boil the bark for the resin or oil they call *yagh*. It is then shipped to Mediterranean trade centers.

SCENT AND APPEARANCE

Its odor is similar to musk and ambergris and is unpleasant in high concentrations. When diluted properly it is reminiscent of the narcissus and tuberose. The gasolinelike top note disappears when the styrene is removed, but it fades anyway with age and blending. Storax is valued more in the East than the West. The Asian variety is preferred but little used in western perfumery.

ASIAN STORAX is viscous or semiliquid, greenish to brownish gray. Water floats on its surface, while heavy particles fall to the bottom. The water-free portion dissolves nearly completely in alcohol. It contains cinnamic acid and ethyl cinnamate, and it varies from the smell of natural storax. Be sure to get a well-cleaned product.

STORAX RESINOID is too impure to use in your blends; it is soluble but produces turbidity. Extraction produces *absolute of storax*, which is olive or greenish brown with a sweet, balsamic odor. Seek purified extract that was not extracted with acetone.

STORAX OIL is steam-distilled from bark. Some materials are represented as this true oil, but they are in fact compounded; price comparisons will tell you which is which. Saponification of bark before steam distillation creates a mild-smelling, neutral material good in florals as a fixative and valued for its mild, balsamic sweetness. It is really natural cinnamic alcohol and is much costlier than the synthetic.

True steam-distilled oil is pale yellow, almost water-white, balsamic, even spicy, with a hint of lilac or hyacinth. But it has the hydrocarbon top note that needs to be leached from the "heads" of the distillate. This styrene note mellows with age.

BLENDING

Storax oil is clearly soluble in all perfumes, and it is inexpensive. Use it with lilac, hyacinth, apple blossom, carnation, cassia, mimosa, violet, hawthorn, lavender, fougere, and rose. Blend it with coumarin, cyclamen, linalool, terpineol, anisaldehyde, ylang-ylang, and jasmine. The spicy note of cinnamic alcohol and cinnamal is exotic and far outlasts the styrene hydrocarbon top note, which dissipates as it polymerizes.

Many so-called storax oils on the market are really cinnamic alcohol, cinnamic esters, or cinnamates with a little vanillin or cinnamal to round them out. Crude types of distillation create natural storax products, but they are not neutral or entirely soluble. Be careful when using these in soap perfumes.

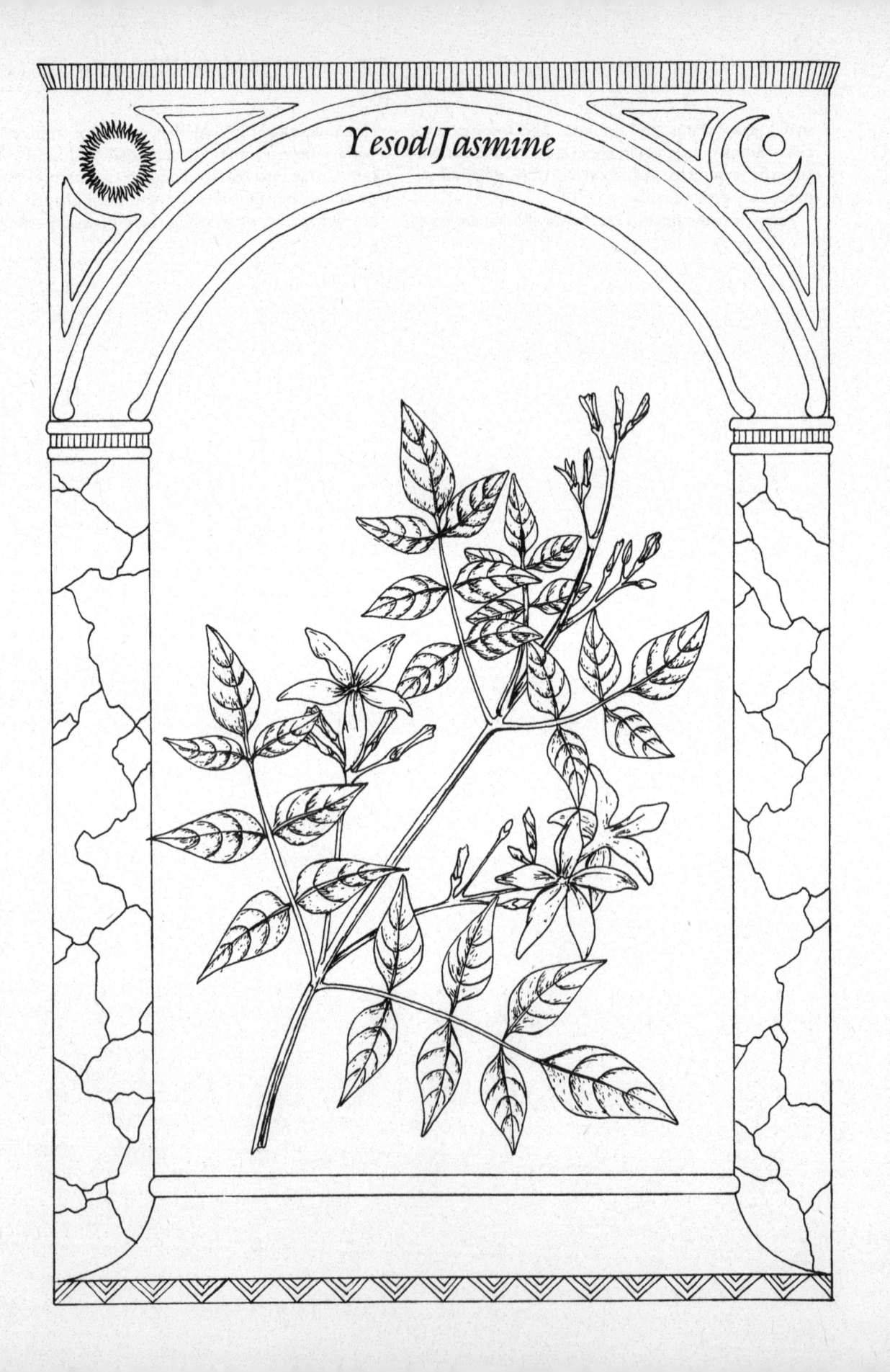

Yesod/Jasmine

> It [jasmine] *is considered second only to the rose in popularity. It was a sacred flower in ancient Persia.*
>
> —Eric Maple, *The Magic of Perfume*

9. YESOD = JASMINE

QABALA

Yesod means Firm Foundation and is associated with the moon. It is the realm of direct experience of the subconscious, as in dreams and imagination. Its symbol is a strong, virile youth; its virginal god-forms include Artemis, Isis, and the White Goddess. Yesod helps us overcome resistance to breaking habits by helping create a new self-image. It relates to harmonious function of the regenerative chakra. Invoke its energies for increased pranic energy. In metaphysics it represents the astral plane, psychism, and trance states. On the psychological level it symbolizes the Jungian concept of anima and animus, the contrasexual aspect of the psyche.

The magical weapons of Yesod are the perfumes and sandals. In *Qabalistic Tarot*, Wang says, "Perfumes suggest its fluid and etheric qualities . . . subtly affecting the minds of the participants. Its qualities are suggestive, yet fleeting and illusory, which is the nature of Yesod." Other qualities and traits of this sphere include dreaminess, fantasy, feelings, fluidity, healing, imagination, impressionability, instincts, loving kindness, memory, motherhood, mystery, purification, rejuvenation, seductiveness, and transformation.

DESCRIPTION

Rose and jasmine, the most important floral notes in perfumery, form the base of a wide range of perfumes. Synthetic jasmine is available, but natural is much sweeter and softer. Even small amounts prove their value. Sometimes ylang-ylang is used to adulterate jasmine.

Oil of jasmine comes from the pure white flowers of *Jasminum grandiflorum* or *Jasminum officinale* or *Jasminum idoranissimum*, natives of India. Oils are obtained by enfleurage (pomade) or solvent extraction. *Jasmine officinale* can grow in any moderate climate, therefore, it is one of the perfumery materials you could grow. Plant it near your bedroom window and the fragrance will waft its way into your room on warm nights from June through autumn.

The perfumes of white and yellow jasmine and *Jasminum sambac* are processed by enfleurage (embedding the petals in fat) and extraction. A thousand plants yield about fifty pounds of flowers per year. Four times this amount is harvested daily during July and August. Jasmine is the most difficult oil to extract and nearly impossible to imitate.

GEOGRAPHIC LOCATION

Originating in India, jasmine is cultivated in most temperate zones. Most of the jasmine available commercially comes from France, Italy, and Egypt, with some grown in Algeria and Morocco. China has a different-smelling species, *Jasminum revolutum*, with yellow flowers, but oil is not produced from it in commercial amounts.

HISTORY

Native to Persia and Kashmir, jasmine was treasured and cultivated early in history. The Persians planted it in their exquisite gardens, according to Xenophon. He spoke of hedges of red roses, white jasmine, and lilacs edged with violets and other delicately scented blooms.

In Indian lore, Kama, god of love, tips his arrows with blossoms to pierce the heart through the senses. One of the scents he fires from his cupid's bow is jasmine, in Arabic *ysmyn*, in Persian *jasemin*.

In China, favored jasmine was strewn on New Year's Day, hung from the eaves of houseboats, put in tea for flavor, and hung in the hair of Chinese girls. Chi Han mentions the wide cultivation of the sambac jasmine Mo Li, from Peking to Canton. In the eighteenth century, Fukien province alone grew more than three million pounds of jasmine. Gardens in Kwangtung province lined the banks of the Pearl River.

An account from 1777 told how the cultivated buds that blossom after dusk are taken to market. Collected at daybreak, clusters of unopened buds were kept wrapped in wet cloth to be sold for use that night, when they opened under the influence of moonlight and body heat. Their romantic scent lingers until dawn.

The Chinese also used jasmine to cleanse a room of the oppressive atmosphere surrounding the sick. Jasmine "balls," probably flowers macerated and mixed with honey, were given to inebriated guests to clear the head of muzziness. It was also used to flavor wine and as a massage oil. Before leaving the lore of the east, it is useful to realize that the so-called red jasmine is actually frangipani, a Philippines plant. Tahitians love this jasmine-scented flower and wear a *tiare* of it in their hair; the word tiara is a corruption of this word.

In the records of Napoleon's perfumer, Chardin, there is a bill for a large bottle of Spanish jasmine, which the Emperor likely bought for Josephine. He preferred eau de cologne. Jasmine reached its height of popularity in the late 1600s when Orange, Genoa, Romane, Frangipani, Neroli, Tuberose, and Marshall were also in vogue. In 1927, Francois Coty introduced L'Aimant, meaning "magnet," a floral bouquet with a jasmine base and a synthetic top note modified with citrus, bergamot, and Bulgarian rose. Another jasmine classic is Lanvin's Arpege, an arpeggio of delicately scented rose, camellia, and lily of the valley.

The poet Edmund Spenser intuitively tapped the link between jasmine and the sexual center in this metaphor about his wife's beauty.

Her breasts, like lilies, 'ere their leaves
  be shed;
Her nipples, like young blossomed
  jessamines;
Such fragrant flowers do give most
  odorous smell
But here sweet odor did them all excel.

SCENT AND APPEARANCE

The notes of jasmine absolutes differ according to their countries of origin. French jasmine is fresh and penetrating. That of Egypt is warmer than the French and languid, coming from a hot country. Italian jasmine combines the qualities of both.

Jasmine concrete de chassis is made from flowers spent during the enfleurage process. Purified, it is used to soften synthetics. The decreasing use of enfleurage have limited the availability.

JASMINE FLORAL ABSOLUTE is extracted from chassis. Rich and tenacious, it shares little else with absolute from concrete. *Jasmine concrete* varies due to processing but is warm and intensely floral, highly diffusive with waxy-herbaceous, oily, fruity, and tealike undertones.

JASMINE ABSOLUTE FROM CONCRETE is the most important extract. A dark orange viscous liquid, its nuances vary from batch to batch.

JASMINE ABSOLUTE FROM POMADE is a product of enfleurage, with a residual fatty off-note from the extraction fat. Its indole note is more pronounced than that of absolute from concrete. All the jasmine fragrances require a lot of handwork in production.

BLENDING

Jasmine absolute rivals rose for rounding off scents. It is so subtle no synthetic jasmines rival the natural fragrance. Perfumers have tried to synthesize jasmine with tealeaf, maté extracts, chamomile and others to no avail. Jasmine bases provide the floral note in eight out of ten floral perfumes. Though expensive, even a minute amount of jasmine absolute more than makes up for its cost.

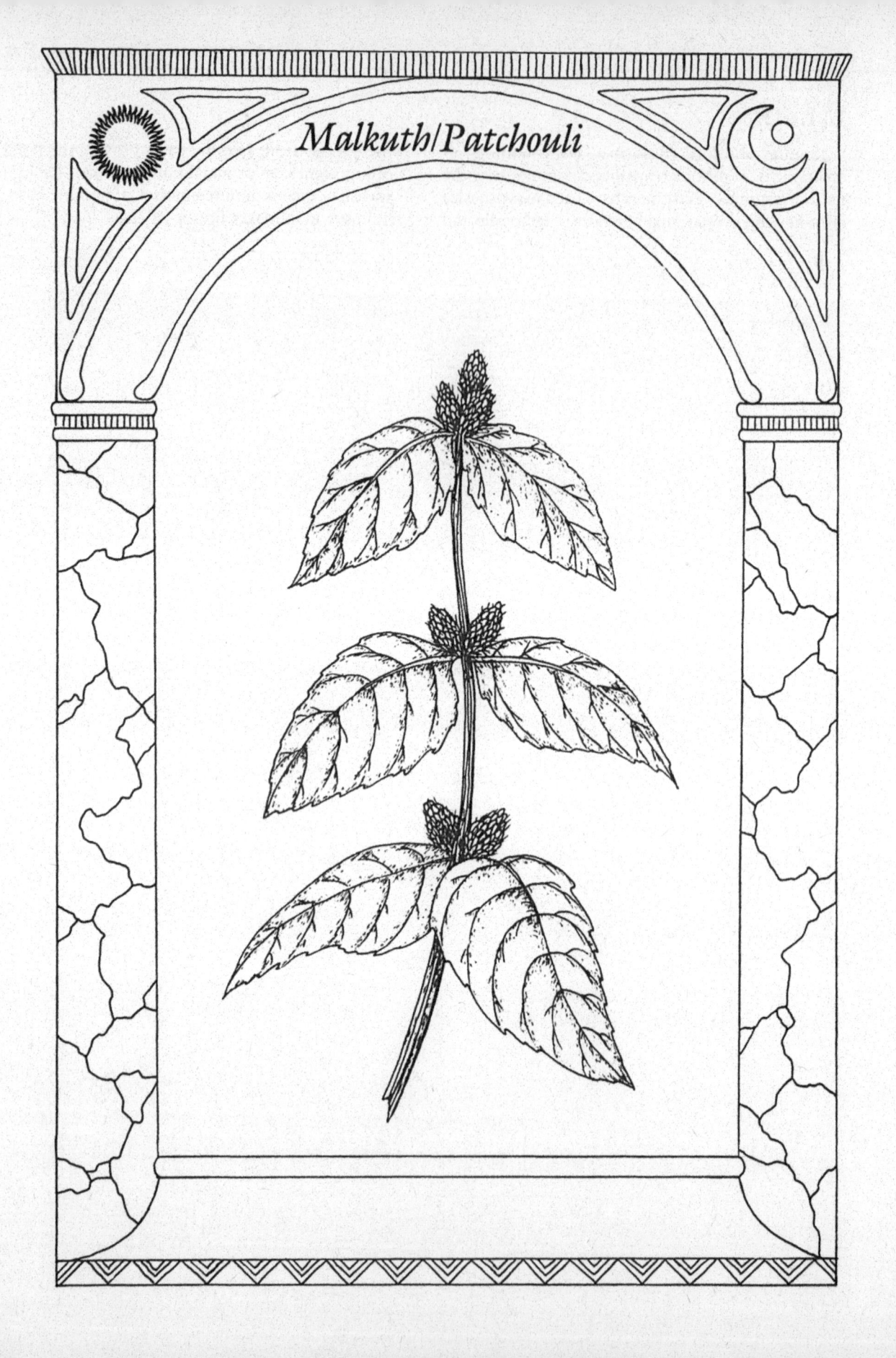

Malkuth/Patchouli

> *Obtained by distilling the dried roots of the oriental plant [patchouli]. . . . It is a fixative of heavy perfumes and also an aphrodisiac with magical powers.*
>
> —Eric Maple, *The Magic of Perfume*

10. MALKUTH = PATCHOULI, DITTANY OF CRETE

QABALA

Malkuth, the Kingdom, represents the earthy sphere of the physical plane. It symbolizes stability and groundedness, but is also the sphere of the beginner in magic, the novice. Its image is a young bride, crowned and throned; she is Persephone or Demeter in myth. The work of Malkuth means resurrecting knowledge of your subconscious complexes. Once you know what they are, your work can begin. They form the blocks or repressions that keep you from evolving.

Malkuth is the sphere of fitness and body work; it also implies a working knowledge of the physical laws of the universe. Purifying the animal drives (survival, lust, hunger) is a requirement for advancement on the Tree of Life. Keywords include earthiness, patience, physical sensation, solid energy, transmutation, and vitality.

Alternates for this sphere include dittany of Crete, *Origanum dictamnus* L., and poppy. Dittany grew in abundance on Mt. Dicte. Its oil is available but its use in ritual was mostly for producing thick smoke for apparitions. William Gray relates earth to poppy, probably because poppy was sacred to Demeter and the intoxicant opium was used in the Elysinian mysteries. Poppyseed oil smells similar to linseed oil, and therefore we feel it is not a sensory equivalent for patchouli.

DESCRIPTION

Patchouli is an important perfume oil distilled from *Pogostemon cablin*. Though evaluations vary, tenacity is characteristic of all patchoulis and adds to its versatility. The leaves of patchouli are ovate, five inches broad and around four inches long. The plant reaches three feet in height, producing whitish flowers sometimes tinged with purple. Oil of patchouli is dark reddish brown with an odor similar to myrrh—a musky sweet heavy odor. Since it is a persistent odor, it makes a great fixative. Its odor improves with age.

GEOGRAPHIC LOCATION

The scent of patchouli became associated with India during the Raj, but it actually originated in the Philippine Islands and Indonesia, where most commercial oil is still produced. The plant is also cultivated in Sumatra, Malaya, the Seychelles, Madagascar, the Chinese coast, and, on a limited basis, in Japan. Indonesian products are distilled in Europe and the United States; they differ greatly from locally distilled oils.

HISTORY

In *The Art of Aromatherapy*, Tisserand recounts the introduction of patchouli to the West, (pp. 262–263):

> Patchouli first became known in Britain about 1820 when it was used to impregnate Indian shawls which became so fashionable that designs were copied by the Paisley weavers for export to many other parts of the world. They

were unable to sell them, however, if not scented with patchouli. In the 1860s patchouli scents enjoyed the same popularity in England as they did in the 1960s. In the East the oil is used to scent linen, and the leaves are used in sachets and pot-pourris.

Patchouli is used in voodoo to bring peace of mind and harmony into the home. Legend says that if it is used to place a hex on someone that hex will boomerang onto the sender.

World production of patchouli has been increasing since 1950 and now exceeds 100 metric tons per year. The price has dropped by about two-thirds since that time, but quality has steadily improved. Since there is an abundance of oil on the market, it is rarely adulterated.

SCENT AND APPEARANCE

When buying patchouli look for two distinct types: native distilled and European or American distilled. Native processed oil is darker, almost brown, while the professional product is a better-refined pale orange or amber color. Native oil is viscous, extremely rich and even sickening in high concentrations. Its sweet-herbaceous, aromatic-spicy, and woody-balsamic odor should have no moldy or musty dry notes. Western oil is also sweet, rich, spicy-aromatic and herbaceous, but it has a top note with a fruity, winelike sweetness and milder woody-earth notes. It can be more spicy-balsamic and even more tenacious than the native oils; it is sweeter.

PATCHOULI RESINOID is a concrete extracted from the dry leaves of patchouli with solvents like benzene or petroleum ether. The syrupy liquid can be further extracted to create an absolute, which yields the heart of the patchouli scent.

BLENDING

Of course, patchouli is frequently the base of oriental blends, but it also goes well with woody bases, fougeres, chypres, opopanax bases, and powder types. Try blending it with labdanum, vetiver, sandalwood, ionones, cedarwood, coumarin, oakmoss, geranium, clove oils, lavender, rose, bergamot, neroli, orris, nitro musks, cinnamates, cassia oil, myrrh, opopanax, clary sage absolute, berneol, and pine needle oils.

Chapter 6

THE ESSENCE OF THE PATHS

On the Tree of Life, the paths connecting the spheres function as a ladder, enabling the aspirant to "climb" the Tree in imagination. The traditional means of active imagining is known as pathworking. From the bottom upward, the twenty-two paths represent the way of return back to union with godhead. In modern terms, pathworking is known as guided visualization or guided imagery, with two main qualifiers: the journey is structured using the symbolism of the path almost exclusively, and the aspirant is expected to actively participate with full moral armament in making any decision in the inner realm.

Pathworking is a magical practice in which the aspirant "journeys" to the imaginal location of an archetypal form for the purpose of communication and acknowledgment. The structure of the pathworking allows the mind to easily locate the archetype in the vast realm within. For example, a pathworking of the thirty-second path begins in Malkuth and travels the Saturn-ruled path to Yesod. This journey would begin on terra firma, move through the universe, culminate at the sphere of the moon, and then return. Symbolism used to set the stage might include gnomes, or a long-bearded old man as a guide (both Saturn symbols); or the White goddess and a gleaming palace of crystal and silver (Moon symbols). The goal is to connect meaningfully with the archetype and anchor the corresponding qualities. Many times this connection is symbolized as a gift, treasure, or embrace.

The paths of the Tree of Life function as metaphorical "in-roads," or means of gaining access to the subconscious. Their correspondences produce an awareness of soul through the Qabala's own system of metaphorical language. Learning this language gives us access to this foreign kingdom. Each successive pathworking increases the area of perceptible inner space. By finding the archetypes in imaginal space the aspirant reconnects with the primordial forces that were called gods and goddesses in ancient times. This connecting provides meaning and empowerment. Be aware that these forces are very powerful and have the capacity to overwhelm a weak ego and disturb the personality. This would be not traveling on an in-road; it would be a premature invasion by the unconscious forces.

The pathworking state is achieved by placing yourself in a light trance by closing your eyes and focusing on your breathing. Calm your mind while relaxing your body and you will soon be approaching the alpha state. Let your cares and worries fall away from awareness, and begin to focus on the opening symbols you have chosen for your path-working.

This exercise of the creative imagination is widely known as astral traveling. In many instances of astral travel, one is compelled in a certain direction; in pathworking the images are not allowed to transform wildly from one to another but are held to a general theme by will. This develops the faculty of clairvoyance, which means seeing the inner world with increasing clarity. This clarity comes through the ego's conscious participation. Clairvoyance is a means of introspection, which connotes looking inside at the stream of interior images.

In pathworking, the will is used to keep the images within certain parameters. The most effective way to do this is to make a script for your excursion and tape it before your pathworking session. You will be able to relax more fully and express your creativity within the format. Normal outward consciousness is turned inward and is brought into direct, nonverbal contact with the irrational. The experience is very enriching. In the spontaneously unfolding scenes there is opportunity to react immediately with feelings or instincts, but remember that you carry the same responsibility for your actions on the inner planes as in the outer.

Pathworking is a preparation for authentic visionary experience. It trains the powers of imagination and concentration and establishes firm relationships with the inner world. Anytime two particular terminals are used, the traveler establishes a contact with the place and the entities found there. With repetition, the imaginal reality of the place is confirmed through personal experience; the aspirant becomes an accepted visitor in that region.

Authentic visionary experience does not require structure, merely a departure point. The free expression of imagery is not a regressive overwhelming by the contents of the lower mind, but an opening and transcendence. The higher mind produces visionary experience with its symbolism of the Way and the higher Self.

The doorway to this type of experience might be a tarot card that corresponds to the paths, an I Ching hexagram, or last night's dream image. The pathworking unfolds spontaneously in those whose visionary imagination transcends active imagining. The visionary imagination creates a crowded canvas of angels and demons, planetary gods, and supercelestial beings. Today we call these figures inner guides and spiritual masters. The practice of pathworking forms a firm foundation for visionary imagination. It provides a medium in which archetypal realities are reflected in the form of vibrant images. It supplies a structure for what is psychically real. It offers an alternative to gross materiality and is a step toward the ultimate sphere of being.

If it seems too overwhelming to construct your own pathworkings, you can find some in books such as *Magical States of Consciousness*, by Denning and Phillips. Gareth Knight's books contain much qabalistic symbolism, as do those of Crowley, and Dion Fortune. Once again, the best way to experience a session is to put it on cassette tape. Listen to the tape with your finger on the pause button, so that you can take all the processing time you need for each scenario.

Anytime you do a pathworking be sure to incorporate the perfume or scent of the path, because this will automatically register the whole gestalt of your experience with your subconscious. Begin your pathworking by using the tarot trump as a door (or perhaps a curtain with the corresponding Hebrew letter on it). Move through the door and find the temple of the sphere you begin in, such as the temple of Malkuth. Build this temple in your imagination with the proper materials, metals, and colors. The surrounding countryside should be appropriate and include all the associated flora and fauna. Consider the atmospheric conditions. Pick a mode of transportation, and begin your journey.

As you continue your journey, leave some imaginal space for the unexpected. Perhaps you will meet a guide or animal or other ally, perhaps there will be challenges or battles. Keep going until you meet with the relevant astrological symbol. Personify this force in a form and try to establish an internal dialogue. When the communication is through, thank this entity for its gifts and communication, then proceed to the temple of the sphere of your destination. Perhaps you are already there. See what awaits you, and then begin your return by the same path back to the point of origin.

It is best to ground these flights of imagination by writing down the result of your excursion as soon as you return to full awareness once again. If you have done your work well, the scent should function thereafter as a very effective anchor for all the qualities and talents you encounter during the pathworking.

> Galbanum *represents the element of Air in that exceedingly powerful incense of Tetragrammaton whose invention is ascribed to Moses.*
>
> —Aleister Crowley, *777*

KEY 11 = THE FOOL = GALBANUM

QABALA

Key #11, Trump 0, Aleph, the Fool, corresponds to the element Air (which represents the Life Breath), the letter A, note E, and the color yellow. This path includes the qualities of spiritual wisdom as well as folly. Further keywords are confidence, divine self, freedom, harmony, holistic health (healing), initiating potential, inner knowing, innocence, joyful aspiration, mastery, mildness, patience, potentiality, questing, superconsciousness, and vitality.

DESCRIPTION

Ferula galbaniflua (Umbelliferae) and other closely related species produce the dried resinous exudation. Coming from five-foot tall, umbrellalike plants, galbanum is an oleoresin containing very little gum. Both hard and soft galbanum are offered commercially, the soft type being used only in perfumery, the other in industry.

GEOGRAPHIC LOCATION

The galbanum-producing plants grow wild in Iran and other parts of Asia Minor, such as Lebanon and Turkey.

HISTORY

Galbanum, which is related to fennel, is mentioned in the Bible in Exodus 20:34. The Greeks, Hippocrates (father of medicine), and Pliny used it. Ecclesiasticus speaks of "a pleasant odor like the best myrrh, as galbanum and onycha." Dr. Hower of Kew Gardens, an expert on plants of the Bible, has identified this as *Ferula galbaniflua*.

SCENT AND APPEARANCE

Soft galbanum, or *levant galbanum*, is dark amber to grayish green or brown. When bought, crude galbanum is viscous and has a gray sludge in the bottom of the container. Poured off from the sludge, the galbanum is refined into oil and resinoids. The odor of the products is woody, green, tenacious, and slightly balsamic or resinous. The green note lends it an airy quality.

GALBANUM OIL is steam-distilled to yield a green, fruity-floral odor reminiscent of green apples, sometimes with a piney top note. Any terpene notes are removed with fractional distillation. The perfumery oil is nearly colorless with an intensely green, leafy odor with a woody undertone. Watch out for galbanum oil tainted with pinene.

GALBANUM RESINOID is extracted, then an odorless solvent is added as a plasticizer to make it pourable. When buying galbanum R. make sure the percentage of solvent is specified. Solvent-free resinoid is also available, as well as a resin absolute, which is alcohol soluble. They are less green and more balsamic and woody than the oil.

BLENDING

Use a modest amount in chypre, fougere, pine, forest, and moss blends, and in florals for a natural leafy character (hyacinth, violet, narcissus, lavender, gardenia). Used in many bases, it blends well with cinnamic alcohol, cyclamal, isoeugenol, linalool, oakmoss, pine, and storax. Resinoid is a good fixative for lavender, fougere, orientals, and woody, mossy types. Its green odor mellows and rounds out synthetics.

> *Mastic is pale yellow and its perfume is singularly clean and free from any prejudice . . . either for or against any particular moral idea. Its action on other perfumes is usually to intensify them and quicken their rate of vibration.*
>
> —Aleister Crowley, *777*

KEY 12 = THE MAGICIAN = MASTIC, STORAX

QABALA

Key #12, Trump I, The Magician, or Magus, is ruled by Mercury, thus sharing the mercurial quality with the sphere of Hod. Its color is orange, letter B, tone E-natural. The perfume storax (or styrax) is also shared by the path and sphere. Therefore, for the qualities of this fragrance, see "Essence of the Spheres," Hod section. Key I (#12 on the Key Scale) expresses the qualities of ability to manifest or actualize, activity, analysis, attention, communication, concentration, creativity, dexterity, energy, initiative, integration, integrity, intelligence, mental activity, persistence, power, psychosynthesis, skill, synthesis, truth, and will.

DESCRIPTION

Mastic, the secondary scent associated with this path, is a natural oleoresin from a small tree of the cashew family, *Pistacia lentiscus* L. The resin in the six-foot high shrubs is harvested by cutting incisions in the bark. The resin solidifies and is collected from June through August. The tears are white or pale yellow, opaque, and about the size of peas. Harvested every fifteen days, a good tree yields eight to ten pounds per season. Tears darken and turn greenish with age. Dry mastic has a faint, balsamic, slightly turpentine odor.

GEOGRAPHIC LOCATION

Indigenous to the Mediterranean coast from Syria to Spain, the shrub also grows in Portugal, Morocco, and the Canary Islands. Most commercial product comes from the Greek island of Chios, just offshore from Izmir in Turkey, and from Cyprus. Small amounts come from Algeria.

HISTORY

The balm mentioned in Genesis as being carried by traders was probably culled from *P. lentiscus*. Known in commerce today as mastic, it has been used for centuries. The Egyptians burned it for incense, while the Jews gave it to their children to chew to strengthen gums and teeth. This is the origin of the word *masticate*. Later, the Greeks flavored a drink made from grapes with it and called this masticke. Do not confuse this with Dammar resin, which is now sold under the name of mastic.

SCENT AND APPEARANCE

Mastic is balsamic with a little turpentine hint. A strong tincture is useful for fixing honeysuckle, lavender, fern, mimosa, and sweet-pea blends. The volatile oil—very scarce and expensive—is pale yellow with a penetrating leafy odor. Resinoid is also available, known in France as *resinoide lentisque*. It is a hard, brittle, pale amber mass, smelling of crude mastic.

BLENDING

Use the oil as a fixative for the above-mentioned blends as well as in citrus colognes, and lavender-fougere. The resinoid is a good fixative which adds a sort of twig odor. In florals it introduces a bitter-woody natural undertone, rounding out the blend. Stellar Visions' formula for this path, known as Beth, includes mastic, calamus, and dill.

> Camphor—*the white waxen appearance suggests Luna, so also the perfume is peculiarly cleanly. Lignum Aloes is a wood in powder, whose physical appearance at once suggests purity of aspiration to the sensitive observer.*
>
> —Aleister Crowley, *777*

KEY 13 = THE HIGH PRIESTESS = CAMPHOR, ALOE

QABALA

Key scale #13, Trump II the High Priestess, is associated with the moon and cool, lunar types of scents. The color of this path is violet; letter G; tone G sharp. The qualities to invoke with these fragrances include association, channeling, psychic experience, mystical experience, purity, meditation, beingness, biorhythms, channeling, devotion, discretion, inner meaning, inspiration, intuition, knowing, love, meditation, memory, mystical experience, polarity, psychic experience, purity, receptivity, reflection, relatedness, revelation, silence, sincerity, soulfulness, spiritual "virginity," suggestibility, support, sympathy, synchronization, and tapping the collective unconscious.

DESCRIPTION

A white, waxy substance, camphor has a penetrating, musty, aromatic smell. The oil comes from the camphor laurel, *Cinnamomum camphora*. Most uses for camphor are industrial, true camphor oil being used only in perfumery. Synthetic camphor, from a-pinene, accounts for half the camphor used in industry.

GEOGRAPHIC LOCATION

Japan and Taiwan produce the best quality camphor-linalool and camphor-safrole type oils. China grows an inferior cineole-terpineol-camphor type.

HISTORY

Valued both for odor and medicinal properties, camphor was known to medieval alchemists, who sometimes confused it with borneo camphor (borneol). In 1833, three chemists (Lavoisier, Boyle, and Dumas) finally analyzed the formula correctly as a compound of carbon, hydrogen, and oxygen.

Cultivated in Taiwan, China, and Japan for centuries, camphor is an important industry there. Camphor is used in fragrance chemistry for soaps as well as cosmetic and medicinal products. In industry it is employed as a flotation agent in mining operations and as a plasticizer and softening agent.

Medicinally, camphor was used in balms as a muscle relaxant. Along with coffee, it is a universal antidote to homeopathic remedies. This property also appears to be known in voodoo, where it is considered a strength-giving body rub and is used to anoint candles.

SCENT AND APPEARANCE

True camphor oil is distilled from the *hon-sho* plant of Taiwan and Japan. The crude oil contains a crystalline mass of crude camphor. Oil is filter-pressed out, yielding crude camphor oil. This is rectified into light, medium, and heavy fractions; only the first two are used for blends. The lightest, white camphor oil, is hardly used except as the raw ingredient for extraction of cineole, pinene, terpineol, menthol, and thymol. Brown camphor oil, the medium fraction, is used to mask unpleasant odors in soap perfumes. It is 80% safrole.

BLENDING

White camphor oil is used to compound synthetic eucalyptus, thyme, rosemary, Spanish sage, and lavandin. It is used in many low-cost household products and disinfectants.

In this pleasant soil
His far more pleasant garden God ordained,
Out of the fertile ground he caused to grow
All trees of noblest kind
  for sight, smell, taste . . .
Laurel and myrtle, *and what higher grew*
Of firm and fragrant leaf: . . .

—Milton, *Paradise Lost*

KEY 14 = THE EMPRESS = SANDALWOOD, MYRTLE

QABALA

Key scale #14 Trump III, the Empress, is associated with Venus or Aphrodite, therefore it partakes of the same essence as Netzach—sandalwood. Its other scent is myrtle. The color of this path is green, its note F sharp, its letter D. Keywords or qualities that convey the positive nature of this path include attraction, beauty, completion, creative imagination, deductive reasoning, delight, desire, elegance, equilibrium, fecundity, fertility, friendship, generation, gentleness, good fortune, graciousness, happiness, harmony, love, luxury, marriage, material wealth, mental images, pleasure, plenitude, rapture, sensuality, trust, understanding, union by enlightenment, vitalization, and wisdom.

DESCRIPTION

Myrtle is the common name for the genus of evergreen shrubs, in particular the highly aromatic *Myrtus communis*, held by the ancients to be sacred to Venus and used as an emblem of love. The plant is generally less than ten feet high with opposite, simple, rather thick and lustrous leaves that are plentifully supplied with minute oil-bearing glands. These glands give the foliage its fragrance. The white or pink solitary flowers are ¾-inch wide, borne on short stalks in the leaf axils. The fruit is purple-black. (Do not confuse with wax myrtle, Oregon myrtle, or California laurel).

GEOGRAPHIC LOCATION

Myrtle is grown in many Mediterranean countries, including Algeria, Corsica, France, Italy, Morocco, Portugal, Sardinia, Spain, Tunisia, Turkey, Yugoslavia, and Cyprus, etc. The shrubs also grow in southern England and the warm parts of the United States.

HISTORY

According to Mohammed, Adam fell down from Paradise with three things: the myrtle, the chief of sweet scented flowers in this world; an ear of wheat, a primary food; and dates, a highly prized fruit.

Greek and Roman folklore alleges that myrtle tea, drunk at least once every three days, has the virtue of preserving love and youth. In love affairs, both parties had to imbibe the drink, which was sometimes mixed with other ingredients to make it more palatable. Woe to the beloved who refused the drink!

SCENT AND APPEARANCE

The essential oil, myrtol, is produced by steam distillation of the leaves, twigs, and sometimes flowers. Batches of oil can vary due to different ratios of ingredients. Distillation is done in France, Corsica, Spain, Italy, Morocco, Tunisia, and Yugoslavia. The oil itself is pale yellow to light amber-colored with a strongly camphoraceous and spicy odor, with sweet-herbaceous and fresh body notes. The best myrtle oils are Tunisian and Corsican. They have very fresh, strong top notes with an almost floral sweetness.

BLENDING

Myrtle oil is used exclusively as a top note. It has no fixative value. Blend it with bergamot, lavandin, lavender, rosemary, clary sage, hyssop, lime oil, and bay. It is a good modifying top note for colognes and aldehydic perfumes. The Stellar Visions blend for the path Daleth is composed of rose, spearmint, and thyme. You might want to try adding just a little myrtle to these other Venusian scents.

With Basil *then I will begin*
Whose scent is wondrous pleasing.

—Drayton, *Polyolbion*

KEY 15 = THE EMPEROR = BASIL

QABALA

Key Scale #15, Trump IV, Tzaddi, the Emperor, is ruled by the fiery zodiacal sign Aries. The letter of the path is H (or E), its color is scarlet, its note C. The attribution is derived from the fact that *basil* is derived from the Greek word for king, *basileus*.

Keywords and qualities stimulated through this path include abundance, achievement, affirmation, ambition, authority, beneficence, confidence, control, duty, expectation, experience, graciousness, helpfulness, kindness, leadership, mental activity, mobility, moral power, overcoming, progression, realization, sanity, self-conquest, self-consciousness, stability, reason, receiving, regeneration, temporal, tenderness, transmitting, triumph, and vision.

DESCRIPTION

Basil oil is distilled from *Ocimum basilicum L.*, also known as common or sweet basil. Basil has a quadrangular stem and dark-green to greyish green leaves 1 inch long and ½ inch wide. It exudes a soft scent of cloves. There are several varieties, but in all of them the flowers appear on spikes. The oil is a limpid yellow with a fresh, penetrating fragrance. Principal ingredients are methyl chavicol with linalool.

GEOGRAPHIC LOCATION

The best oils come from Cyprus and the Seychelles, but the herb is grown commercially in Europe, North Africa, and Reunion (an island east of Madagascar).

HISTORY

Basil was considered a royal herb because, as Parkinson says, "the smell thereof is so excellent that it is fit for a king's house." It may have been used in some royal healing balm or unguent. In Crete, basil symbolized "love washed with tears," and it is still used in Italy as a love token. In Moldavia, folklore holds that anyone taking a sprig of the plant from a maiden will fall in love with her. In India, this plant, held sacred to Krishna and Vishnu, is placed on the breasts of the dead as their passport to paradise.

SCENT AND APPEARANCE

There are two types of basil oil: (1) sweet basil oil, a linalool type, distilled mainly in France and America, and (2) the exotic or Reunion oil, which is a camphor-estragole type. Sweet basil oil contains no camphor, is pale yellow to colorless, and is expensive, due to low production. Its smell is sweet-spicy, slightly green, with a long-lasting sweetness and woody undertone.

The exotic oil is yellow to pale green in color, smells more herbaceous and camphoraceous, with an intense sweetness akin to anise. It is cheaper but does not replace the French type oil. Exotic oil is sometimes cut with linalool and called French.

There are also methylcinnamate and phenolic types of basil oil from other countries and species.

BLENDING

Sweet basil oil is a classic ingredient in the origan types, chypres, aldehydic, and green perfume blends. Use it with opoponax, bergamot, isoeugenol, clary sage, lime oil, oakmoss, and citrus oils. Exotic oil is really only suitable for low-cost perfumes, such as those for soap. Stellar Visions' blend includes the Mars-ruled scents coriander, pine, and basil.

> *Perhaps no plant of the New World has been more widely used in perfumery ... than the vanilla. ... It was Professor Johnson who stated that, physiologically, the scent of vanilla acts upon the system as an aromatic stimulant, exhilarating the mental functions, and increasing generally the energy of the animal system.*
>
> —Genders, *Perfume Through the Ages*

KEY 16 = THE HIEROPHANT = STORAX, VANILLA

QABALA

Key scale #16, Trump V, the Hierophant, is related to earthy Taurus. This sign, ruled by the planet Venus, has traditionally been ascribed to the more mercurial storax. Despite its sweetness, vanilla allegedly also stimulates the mental function symbolized here. This path's letter is V (or U), color is red-orange, tone C sharp. An exalted aspect of devotion is represented by this path, that of earthly man for the sweet divine.

Qualities of the Hierophant we seek to integrate include the following: alliance, benediction, conscience, consecration, constructive energy determination, endurance, goodness of heart, groundedness, inspiration, interior hearing, intuition, meditation, organization, patience, peace, placidity, purification, religious inspiration, serenity, strength, teaching, and temperance.

DESCRIPTION

Fine oil comes from the unripe pods of *Vanilla planifolia Andr*. This orchid is a climbing vine that bears flowers. It is cultivated by placing yard-long vine cuttings in soil at the bottom of tall trees. Flowers are greenish yellow; pods are about nine inches long and are gathered in September. Covered with crystals of vanillin, they are termed frosted.

GEOGRAPHIC LOCATION

Native to tropical forests of Brazil and Mexico, the orchid is cultivated in Bourbon, Madagascar, Tahiti, and Java.

HISTORY

Since its discovery, vanilla was widely used until the synthesizing of vanillin from coal tar in 1875. The pods were first imported to England at the end of the sixteenth century. An apothecary showed one he had gotten from Spanish merchants to Elizabeth I. The pods were sliced and soaked in alcohol to prepare a tincture.

SCENT AND APPEARANCE

Perfumery products include vanilla absolute, vanilla extracts of varying concentrations, a resinoid, and a tincture. The absolute lacks the total aroma of the crude fruit, is dark brown with a rich, sweet odor, and is semisolid. In perfume, the extracts are often substituted for by absolute. Vanilla tincture for perfumery is made with perfume alcohol and differs in composition from that for flavoring. Perfume tincture runs about 10% vanilla in 95% alcohol.

BLENDING

Vanilla adds richness and depth to sweet florals, amber bases, and oriental perfumes; it blends well with sandalwood, vetiver, opoponax, and spice oils. True vanilla is very tenacious, with a uniform dryout. Stellar Visions' blend for the path Vau includes earthy patchouli, sweet vanilla, and myrtle—sacred to Venus, which rules Taurus.

> Wormwood *probably pertains to Gemini on account of the intellectual stimulation which it affords in such a magical preparation as Absinthe.*
>
> —Aleister Crowley, *777*

KEY 17 = THE LOVERS = WORMWOOD

QABALA

Key scale #17, Trump VI, the Lovers, is ruled by Gemini; its letter is z, color orange, musical note D. In attributing wormwood to this path because of the mental effects it causes when ingested, Crowley seems to have overlooked the psychosensory effects of the pure fragrance. Though we will cover wormwood here, other sources suggest alternatives such as mastic, bay, lavender, or orchid, which aptly capture the essence of the Lovers.

The qualities we seek to invoke along this path include accomplishment, discrimination, adaptation, divine guidance, bhakti (devotion or adaptation), beauty, devotion, discipleship, discrimination, divine guidance, harmony, inspiration, love, intuition, resolution, symbiosis, synthesis of consciousness and unconsciousness, temptation.

DESCRIPTION

Wormwood oil is steam-distilled from the dried herb (leaves and flowering tops of the plant) *Artemesia absinthium*, known in the United States as mugwort. It should not be confused with the Chinese so-called mugwort, which is a different species. Wormwood is used to flavor vermouth, along with angelica root, anise seed, and marjoram.

GEOGRAPHIC LOCATION

A native of central and southern Europe, where it grows wild in abundance, wormwood is also cultivated in France, Holland, Belgium, Germany, the southeastern Soviet Union, North Africa, and Brazil. It is also a common weed in Oregon, Michigan, Indiana, and Wisconsin.

HISTORY

There is an English recipe for a love philtre dating from the 1400s, which perhaps links this herb to the Lovers. This rather gruesome spell includes using the left index finger of a hanged man—the finger is cut while the body is still warm and swinging aloft. (Fortunately, these are somewhat hard to come by these days.) The finger is cut, mixed with wormwood, and served to the beloved. The powerful vibrations of this tasty morsel are supposed to ensure potency, and apparently, prolong the sweet agonies of love. The agony might only be in eating the philtre!

Wormwood oil is made from the same plant used to concoct the narcotic drink, absinthe, popular in France during the impressionist period. The drink, containing a toxic narcotic, thujone, was banned in 1915.

SCENT AND APPEARANCE

Wormwood oil is very dark green to bluish colored with an intensely herbaceous, green, warm, deep odor, with a fresh top note somewhat like cedar oil. The tenacious body note is warm and dry-woody. Variations in odor come from wormwood oil fractions, which isolate the more interesting notes, especially the intensively green-herbaceous note, the dry-woody note, and a sweet, leathery note. The thujone is boiled off, hence the oil has no mind-altering quality.

BLENDING

Partially "de-thujonized" wormwood oil blends well with oakmoss, as a herbaceous note in jasmine, orange flower, or hyacinth; it lends a richness to chypre and lavender. Wormwood oil adds life and warmth to modern fantasy bases, particularly with oakmoss. Wormwood absolute is hard to come by. Stellar Visions' blend for Zain is based on mastic, bay, and lavender.

After diligent reflection on all these diverse options, there is little doubt in my mind that onycha of Exodus 30:34 is labdanum . . . it is not only ideally suited for use in incense, but it is also a product of the Jewish homeland.

—Harold J. Abrahams, in *Economic Botany*, 33(2), 1979

KEY 18 = THE CHARIOT = ONYCHA (LABDANUM)

QABALA

Key scale #18, Trump VII, Cheth the Chariot, is ruled by the lunar sign, Cancer. Cancer's traditional scent, onycha has been traced by scholars to be labdanum, a rock rose. Another alternate scent is lotus. The letter of this path is Ch; its color orange-yellow; musical note D sharp. Qualities of this path you may wish to integrate include appraisal, attention, audacity, conquest of illusion, faithfulness, hope, inner mystery, master-power, memory, obedience, perfection, perseverance, receptivity, refinement, renunciation, steadfastness, success, triumph, victory, volition, and zeal.

DESCRIPTION

Labdanum is a resinous exudate collected from the shrub *Cistus ladaniferus* (Cistaceae). The whole plant is steam distilled. Products obtained by other processes include concrete, resinoid, resinoid absolute, and resin absolute. All are slightly different, but generally their odor is balsamic, floral, pleasant, and ambered. The Cretan quality is finest and more ambered than the rest. Crude labdanum is imported in brownish or greenish lumps, contaminated with hair and broken leaves.

GEOGRAPHICAL LOCATION

The shrub is widely distributed over the rocky ground of Macedonia, Thrace, Greece, southern France, Spain, Portugal, northern Africa and the islands of Crete and Cyprus, where it grows in abundance. Rock rose likes the mountainous coastal regions of eastern Mediterranean countries and the Middle East.

HISTORY

Onycha has been the subject of great controversy, having been listed in the Bible as an ingredient in the temple incense of Moses. In fact, this is the first written recipe for a perfume, given in Exodus 30:34, which reads:

> And the Lord said unto Moses, Take unto thee sweet spices, stacte and onycha, and galbanum; these sweet spices with pure frankincense: of each there shall be a like weight: and thou shalt make it a perfume, a confection after the art of the apothecary, tempered together, pure and holy: and thou shall not make to yourselves according to the composition thereof: it shall be unto thee holy for the Lord.

A widely accepted theory of its origin was that it came from the small mollusk *Strombus lentiginosus*, found on the shores of the Red Sea; from it a fragrant essence was obtained. Others identified it as *Unguis odoratus*. Crowley fell for the "onycha as mollusk" argument and, thinking it was a shellfish, attributed it to the watery path of Cancer.

Abrahams, in "Onycha, Ingredient of the Ancient

Jewish Incense: An Attempt at Identification," brings up an irrefutable point in this controversy:

> The widely held mollusk hypothesis becomes quite perplexing if one considers that the mollusk was counted among the unclean animals in the Bible. . . . It seems highly unlikely that the use of the mollusk or of parts of the mollusk was intended or permitted for rites in the Holy Tabernacle, and this is indeed confirmed by the famed theologian Nachmanides, who emphasized that the commandment concerning unclean animals pertained not only to dietary rules, but to the temple service as well.

Abrahams sides with the renowned Arabic scholar and writer Saadya (882–942), born in upper Egypt and educated in Old Cairo. He translated the Bible into Arabic. Equally versed in Hebrew, Greek, and Arabic, he knew the people and customs of the whole region intimately. Saadya's translation for *shecheleth*—the Hebrew term—was the Arabic *ladana*, our ladanum or labdanum.

In Cyprus, labdanum was collected from the fleeces of sheep, which acquired the sticky resin while grazing. From May to July the oleoresin is very glutinous. Leather thongs, called *ladanisterion*, are used for collection today in Crete and Cyprus. Resin is scraped from the thongs with a knife, then purified.

SCENT AND APPEARANCE

The finest labdanum product in perfumery is true cistus oil, distilled from the whole herb. It is a pale orange-colored liquid with a warm-herbaceous odor, somewhat like Roman chamomile or decaying fruit. Oil from the herb is inferior in tenacity to oil from gum labdanum, its power is in its top note. Purified gum resin is either yellowish brown or green with a powerful but sweet characteristic odor, somewhat like ambergris, with excellent fixative properties. Labdanum yields between 1% and 2% volatile oil.

BLENDING

Labdanum is important because it resembles ambergris and is cheaper than that essence. Use it to fix lavender, fern, chypre, verbena, and violet types and to round out artificial ambers. Cistus oil is good for colognes and lavender bouquets. Labdanum absolute is used in citrus colognes, lavender colognes, oriental bases, chypres, amber bases, pine, and forest blends. Use them with nitro musks, oakmoss, clary sage, bergamot, lavender, calamus, lavandin, citrus oils, and opoponax. Stellar Visions combines the lunar jasmine with lemon and nard for a Cheth essence.

> Olibanum, *combining the ideas of fire and Sol, is pre-eminently suited for Leo, the Kerub of Fire, the house of the Sun.*
>
> —Aleister Crowley, *777*

KEY 19 = STRENGTH/LUST = OLIBANUM

QABALA

Key scale #19 is Trump VIII, known alternatively, as Strength or Lust. It corresponds to the sign Leo, which is under the rulership of the sun. Its letter is T, color yellow, musical note E sharp. This path symbolizes action, balance of severity and mercy, compassion, compensation, courage, energy, faith, fortitude, initiation, intuition, kundalini, might, moral force, organization, power, profundity, rapture, responsibility, and vigor. Its traditional essence is olibanum or frankincense, which is used to bless, protect, cleanse, and consecrate and to attract success and prosperity.

SCENT

For further information on olibanum, see Sphere 6, Tiphareth. Other oils that come under the rulership of the Sun can be used for blending with olibanum oil for essences that express Strength. Stellar Visions' excellent blend includes cinnamon, olibanum, and nutmeg.

Other solar oils include the following: acacia, angelica, azalea, bay, chamomile, cassia, eucalyptus, galangal, heliotrope, marigold, passionflower, peony, rosemary, and saffron.

Narcissus *refers to the solitary tradition* . . .

—Aleister Crowley, *777*

KEY 20 = THE HERMIT = NARCISSUS

QABALA

Key scale #20, Trump IX, Yod, is governed by the sign Virgo, hence the planet Mercury. Its letter is Y (or I or J), its color is yellow-green, and note F. On this path the desirable qualities and attributes we seek to connect with include affection, attainment, caution, circumspection, council, detachment, discretion, enlightenment, faithfulness, foresight, intelligence, meditation, patience, responsiveness, retreat, secrecy, selectivity, the Self, silence, tuning in, union of opposites, uplift, Wise Old Man archetype, and withdrawal. An alternative scent is that of the lily, a plant attribute of this path. The madonna lily especially recalls the virginal nature of this path.

DESCRIPTION

From the daffodil family, *Narcissus poeticus* is the source of absolute oil of narcissus. The absolute is extracted from a concrete made with volatile solvent. The absolute is dark greenish brown to dark yellow.

GEOGRAPHIC LOCATION

Cultivated as an ornamental in North America, narcissus is also widespread and cultivated in the south of France, especially the valleys of the Cevennes. There are two types of absolute: the narcissus cultivated on the plains of Grasse and the mountain type, which is that of Cevennes and the hills near Grasse. It is also cultivated in Holland.

HISTORY

The name *narcissus* is not derived from the Greek youth who gazed at his reflection, but from the Greek word *narkao*, meaning "to benumb." Its poisonous and narcotic properties led to its consideration as a portent of death. It functioned this way in the myth of the abduction of Persephone by Hades, Lord of Death. She was picking narcissus flowers when Hades seized her to make her his bride and queen of Hades. According to the Homeric hymn, Persephone was . . .

picking flowers,
roses, and crocus
and beautiful violets,
in lush meadow,
and iris, and hyacinth,
narcissus even
which Earth,
as a trick,
   grew
for this girl
as a favor for
Him Who Receives So Many
From its root
it pushed up
a hundred heads
and a fragrance
from its top
   making
all the vast sky above
   smile,

and all the earth,
and all the salt swelling
of the sea.
—*The Homeric Hymns*, Charles Boer, trans.

The Arabians extolled this oil as an aphrodisiac and a cure for baldness.

SCENT AND APPEARANCE

Narcissus absolute is a sometimes grainy, viscous liquid. Its odor is strongly foliage green, very sweet-herbaceous with a faint but lasting floral undertone. It has moderate tenaciousness. *Des plains* oil, from Grasse, is orange-colored with a floral, sweet, mild, and rich odor that is not very powerful. *Des montagnes*, on the other hand, is greenish brown with a powerful, sharp, green, earthy odor, with a hint of violet leaves. It has a sweet, floral, but still green undertone.

BLENDING

Production is limited, so use of the absolute is limited. Blends well with clove bud absolute, carnation, jasmine, orange flower, ylang-ylang, rose de mai, and mimosa. Synthetic narcissus blends use cinnamic alcohol, ionone, eugenol, and other chemicals rounded off with ylang-ylang and tuberose. Well-known perfumes with the narcissus note are Narcisse Noir of Caron, the Narcisse Bleu of Mury, and Que Sais-je by Patou. Absolute is usually "bouqueted" with violet, mimosa, and indole. For Yod, Stellar Visions recommends mastic, olibanum, and bergamot.

Forms are the vases into which I pour
The precious perfume of mine inmost essence,
And where I am,
There must truth and right abide.

—Paul Foster Case, "The Meditation on Kaph,"
The Book of Tokens

KEY 21 = THE WHEEL OF FORTUNE = SAFFRON

QABALA

Key scale #21, Trump X, Kaph, is blue in color; its note is A sharp, and letter K. Kaph, the Wheel of Fortune, is the symbol of the initiate, showing that the sorrowful, weary wheel of unconscious life has been transmuted. Thus one leaves the state of unconscious relationship with the Self and relates to a different wheel of conscious relationship. This is expressed in the Orphic philosophy of the Roman philosopher Porphyry: "I have passed with eager feet to the Circle desired." The circle desired is a more conscious one, with the Lord of Fortune as rewarder and conciliator. The Greek word here translated as "circle" also means "crown." This relates to this Jupiter path as the image of a philosopher king. Ritual crowning used in initiation has to do with proclaiming wholeness by composing the circle, or wheel.

Qualities associated with this path are ambition, arrogance, benevolence, conciliation, dynamism, energy, enthusiasm, exactitude, expansion, extraversion, fortune, independence, leadership, lucky, magnificence, nobility, optimism, power, prosperity, respect, restlessness, self-assurance, wholeness, and wisdom.

DESCRIPTION

Saffron comes from the dried stylus of the flower, *Crocus sativus*, cousin of the garden crocus. Saffron oil is not commercially available. Even if it were, saffron is one of the most expensive botanical raw materials and so the oil would be quite expensive.

GEOGRAPHIC LOCATION

Saffron originated in western Asia, Asia Minor, and the eastern Mediterranean but is also cultivated in Spain, Turkey, Greece, Persia, India, and the Soviet Union.

HISTORY

Known to the Jews as *karcom* (Song of Solomon 4:14), the crocus was also used by the Greeks and Romans. Even after saffron was imported to England from the East, its price remained high, since it takes 60,000 flower stigmas to make one pound of saffron; 4,320 flowers produce only one ounce of crude saffron.

Saffron was cultivated in Persia as early as the tenth century. It is from the Arab *zaffer* that the word *saffron* is derived. Used as a dye in Eastern Asia, saffron's yellow color was considered to symbolize perfection. The Greeks also admired its color, but they valued the scent just as highly.

SCENT AND APPEARANCE

Dried stigmas have a peculiar, intensely sweet, spicy, floral-aldehydic smell with an underlying fatty herbaceousness because of the aldehyde, safranal. Since commercial oil is not available consumers must produce tinctures according to their needs.

Essential oil can be produced; it is pale yellow with a strong odor, but it is extremely unstable. Instead, prepare a concentrated 20% tincture from saffron with diluted alcohol over gentle heat.

BLENDING

Add minute amounts to violet perfumes, narcissus, and neroli bases. Saffron adds great interest to oriental blends. Since it is expensive or difficult to acquire this product, you may prefer to use other traditional Jupiter-related scents such as cedar, nutmeg, and clove.

Mint Bouquet Oil: *Removes bad spells.*

—Robert W. Pelton, *The Complete Book of Voodoo*

KEY 22 = ADJUSTMENT = GALBANUM, MINT

QABALA

Key scale #22, Trump XI, Adjustment, corresponds with Libra, Venus, the color green; letter l; and tone F sharp. It signifies balance, justice, and equilibrium. The main scent of this path is the airy galbanum. Others attribute both peppermint and spearmint to this Venus-ruled sign. Justice is a duality combining moral force with constructive purpose, yielding great achievement. Its virtues include compensation, consistency, decisiveness, discernment, ecology, integrity, judgment, law and order, ordinance, partnership, poise, regulation, reward/punishment, and a strong sense of duty. This path is also related to the law of karma, of which Pythagoras says in his *Golden Verses:*

> Carefully consider before you act.
> You may not be able to retract.
> Understand well all that you do
> And you will have no cause to rue.

DESCRIPTION

Spearmint oil comes from *Mentha spicata*; peppermint oil from *Mentha piperita*. Mints have square stalks, and the perennial spreads by underground, creeping roots. The main constituent of spearmint oil is carvone; peppermint contains menthol.

GEOGRAPHIC LOCATION

Native to the Mediterranean area of Europe, it has spread to the United States. It is cultivated widely in Hungary, the Soviet Union, and the United States.

HISTORY

The synonyms of spearmint show it has been revered as Our Lady's mint (menthe de Notre Dame to the French), and sage of Bethlehem. The Romans and Greeks cultivated it extensively and Pliny and Ovid wrote of it. In ancient Israel tithes were paid in mint, anise, and cumin. Widely used in Athens, it was rubbed on the arms in particular, probably as a powerful deodorant. In medieval times it was used for strewing on floors and later to overcome tobacco odors. The Greeks and Romans used crowns of peppermint to adorn themselves for festive occasions. Peppermint oil is used ritually to clear the mind and calm the nerves while attracting the good things of life.

SCENT AND APPEARANCE

Spearmint oil is steam-distilled from the flowering tops of the plants. The pale yellow- to olive-colored oil smells warm and slightly herbaceous, with the characteristic powerful, penetrating mint odor.

Peppermint, known to practically everyone, is hardly used in perfumery. The oil is pale yellow to olive with a deeply sweet, balsamic undertone and a sweet, refreshing dryout. A grassy top note fades as the oil ages. The odor gives the same immediate psychological impression of coolness associated with the flavor and aroma.

BLENDING

Spearmint oil is used in green perfumes (note the green color of this path) as well as in lavender-fougere, and jasmine compositions. Carvone blends nicely with jasmine. Peppermint oil can be used in lavender colognes for lift and freshness as well as in fougeres and geranium bases. Small quantities of mint oils give character to a compatible perfume. Stellar Visions' blend for Lamed includes cypress, galbanum, and spearmint.

> Myrrh Oil: *A powerful aid to ward off evil and to break hexes. Popular for uncrossing friends.*
>
> —Robert Pelton, *The Complete Book of Voodoo*

KEY 23 = THE HANGED MAN = ONYCHA, MYRRH

QABALA

Key scale #23, Trump XII, the Hanged Man, is the path of elemental water. Its letter is M; color blue; tone G sharp. This path connects the personality with the higher Self through self-sacrifice and redemption. It also is the suspension of sensory awareness that comes during higher consciousness. Its qualities and keywords include baptism, enforced sacrifice, impressionability, intuition, moodiness, possessiveness, potency, prophetic powers, prudence, spirituality, and wisdom.

SCENT

These fragrances are covered extensively under "Binah" and "The Chariot." Try various combination of cistus oil and myrrh for the path of Mem. Myrrh has been long used as a sacred oil for blessing and protection. It also aids meditation and promotes healing.

> *Opoponax refers even more directly to Scorpio than does Siamese Benzoin. There is in it even less of the sensuousness of pleasure; there is an overpowering richness of the deliciously abominable.*
>
> —Aleister Crowley, *777*

KEY 24 = DEATH = BENZOIN, OPOPONAX

QABALA

Key scale #24, Trump XIII, Death, is attributed to Scorpio, which is ruled by Mars. Its letter is N; color blue-green; note G. This path does not necessarily literally indicate death, rather, the death of the old self, or an outmoded condition. It is transformation of energy, a change in the form of consciousness, or rebirth after ego-death. Nun also signifies ascension to a higher realm. Its keywords include competition, creativity, destruction and renewal, detachment, hypnosis, imagination, impulsiveness, liberation, movement, putrefaction, readjustment, regeneration, recycling, rejuvenation, resurrection, transformation, and unselfishness. A third alternative scent is pine.

DESCRIPTION

A perennial with a thick, fleshy root, opoponax grows from 1 to 3 feet high with branching stems. The flowers are yellowish and grow in flat umbels. Oleoresin is harvested by cutting into the base of the stem. This produces tears, or small irregular pieces of reddish-yellow color, covered with white specks. Opoponax comes from *Commiphora erythroea*.

GEOGRAPHIC LOCATION

This medium-sized tree, related to myrrh, comes from Somaliland, eastern Africa, and eastern Ethiopia, but the resin is only collected in Somaliland.

HISTORY

Opoponax is also known as bisabol, perfumed bdellium, and sweet myrrh. In magic it is used for protection and purification. In Somalia it is called *habbak hadi*—gum of the haddit tree. The Chinese use it in religious worship. The original so-called opoponax of ancient times probably came from *Balsamodendron kafal* or *kataf*, of Sudan and Arabia. This product has been replaced because of the superior floral-amber character of the *Commiphora* species.

SCENT AND APPEARANCE

The crude botanical product is dark reddish tears, with a smell reminiscent of myrrh but with spicy, animal, rootlike overtones. It is not as light and fresh as myrrh. The oil is steam-distilled from selected raw material. It is pale yellow to orangish, even somewhat olive- or amber-colored. It is intensely sweet, balsamic, warm, and spicy, smelling somewhat of wine dregs. Watch for adulteration with myrrh oil, lovage, pine needle fraction, or copaiba balsam. Opoponax resinoid is hydrocarbon-extracted and has a plasticizer added. It is an excellent fixative when its dark color is not a deterrent.

BLENDING

The oil blends with clary sage; coriander; labdanum; woody and floral perfumes; chypre; fougere, leather, and oriental bases; bergamot; nitro musks; patchouli; mimosa; fir needle absolute; and neroli oil. Resinoid is warm and powdery—good for Orientals and for spicy effects in forest blends, moss notes, and heavy florals. Opoponax anydrol has certain of the notes but is nearly colorless. Stellar Visions' blend for Nun includes musk, pine, and violet.

> *The perfume of* Lignum Aloes *intuitively suggests horsemanship in an airy racecourse.... It is therefore to Sagittarius ... as the path leading from Yesod to Tiphareth, that this perfume applies.*
>
> —Aleister Crowley, *777*

KEY 25 = TEMPERANCE/ART = ALOE

QABALA

Key scale #25, Samekh, Trump XIV, Art, corresponds to Sagittarius, the letter S; color blue, and the tone G sharp. This path refers to the dissolution of old patterns and reformation of the personality through psychoanalysis. It means precise balancing of the opposites of positive and negative, creating a divine synthesis. This path is related to personal consecration, creating a magical link between the mundane and divine. Its traits and qualities include abandon, androgyny, chastity, courage, dedication, devotion, dignity, diligence, fiery zeal, flexibility, frankness, harmony, independence, mutability, oscillation, philosophicality, restlessness, undomesticatedness, and unselfishness.

DESCRIPTION

Aloe is the commonly used term for agar oil. *Aquilaria agallocha* is the source of the tree's fungus-infected wood, which is distilled for the odoriferous oil. Lign-aloe is totally different from medicinal aloe, such as *aloe vera*, which originated in Africa. Lign-aloe is a corruption of the Latin *lignum-aloes*—and is thus a type of wood rather than a resin.

GEOGRAPHIC LOCATION

These plants are cultivated in northeastern India and certain parts of China. Both wood and oils can be difficult to obtain, not being listed in any buyer's directories.

HISTORY

Aloes are mentioned in the Bible in Proverbs 7:17: "I have perfumed my bed with myrrh, aloes, and cinnamon." The term *aloe-wood* is used in India to signify many fragrant woods. True agar wood has been known and used perhaps as long as sandalwood. Lign-aloe is also referred to in the Bible in Numbers 24:6. Dioscorides refers to *agallochon* as a wood imported from Arabia or India. He noted that it was odoriferous, with an astringent or bitter taste. The traditional magical use is for protection and healing. Sadi, a Persian poet, described aloes:

> The aloes-wood, from which no fragrance came,
> If placed on fire, its inodorous state
> Will change, more sweet than ambergris.

SCENT AND APPEARANCE

Fungus-infected trees produced the oleoresin, which is then distilled under pressure. Agar oil ranges from pale yellow to dark amber. This very viscous liquid is sweet and rich with a woody-balsamic note and a sweetness reminiscent of sandalwood. Agar oil is only produced for firm orders.

BLENDING

If you can find agar oil; use it for orientals, woody-aldehydic bases, fougeres, and in sandalwood and linalool mixtures. Stellar Visions substitutes other Jupiterian scents such as cedar, hyssop, and dill.

> Musk *and* Civet *are referred here on account of their sexual origin, and of their effect upon the aura of the magician. The regular Saturnian perfumes would only be employed in malefic work and in other baser aspects of Capricorn.*
>
> —Aleister Crowley, *777*

KEY 26 = THE DEVIL = MUSK, CIVET (BAY)

QABALA

Key scale #26, Trump XV, the Devil, is Capricorn; letter O; color violet; tone A. This path represents the test against the temptation to use spiritual powers for personal gain or gross sensuality, the downward pull of instinctuality. It is a line of direct contact between the higher Self and personality. It leads from the use of intellect to intuition. This path makes us aware of our misperceptions of reality. Since the Saturnian scents are for malefic work, we suggest the solarscent, bay, which is traditionally used to counteract negativity, ward off evil, and stimulate psychic vision. Keywords and qualities include excitation, instinctuality, lustiness, spontaneity, and overcoming handicaps.

DESCRIPTION

Bay oil is distilled from the leaves of *Myrcia acris*. The bay oil from the California bay laurel or Oregon myrtle is called myrtlewood oil and is different from the oil of the Venusian shrub. Five-year-old trees are harvested in the dry months, yielding 60 to 100 pounds of leaves annually.

GEOGRAPHIC LOCATION

The source for *Myrcia acris* is the West Indies, for *Lauris nobilis*, the Pacific coast of the United States.

HISTORY

Sweet bay was used to crown Greek poets, heroes, and victors, particularly in the ancient Olympic Games. In the Middle Ages it was employed in various rituals to prevent evil and was prized for alleged medicinal value. It was known as Daphne to the Greeks and considered sacred to Apollo.

SCENT AND APPEARANCE

Terpenless bay leaf oil is pale and straw-colored to brown or orange. It is steam-distilled after the turpentine is removed or alcohol-washed. It is intensely sweet, deep, and mellow with spicy-balsamic notes. It has a lemony top note and is soluble in alcohol.

BLENDING

Use it with lavandin or lavender, petitgrain, citrus oils, rosemary, geraniol, cinnamic alcohol, and ylang-ylang for many perfume bases. Stellar Visions combines it with wormwood and cypress to preserve the Saturnian quality of the path Ayin yet keep it positively oriented.

> Pepper *is evidently Martial owing to its fiery quality and its specific action on the mucous membrane of the nostrils.... Heat and pungency are two principal qualities of Mars.*
>
> —Aleister Crowley, 777

KEY 27 = THE TOWER = PEPPER

QABALA

Key scale #27, Trump XVI, the Tower, is ruled by Mars, with the letter P; tone C; and color red. The pungent and caustic nature of pepper reflects the nature of this path, which signifies the startling awakening of superconsciousness that can come as a shock as well as a clear flash of vision. The breakdown of the fortress of the personality opens one to the establishment of the divine. This path is the balancing of reason with desire. This inner growth can sometimes be painful and even overwhelming. There are positive and negative traits on this path, some to acquire and some to transmute: anger, bravery, brutality, courage, defensiveness, discipline, dissipation, dominance, impetuosity, impulsiveness, irritability, maliciousness, militance, obstinance, strength, valor, vehemence, vigor, volatility, and zeal.

DESCRIPTION

From the immature fruits of the pepper vine, *Piper nigrum*, black pepper oil is steam distilled; so-called Lampong pepper is preferred for perfume oil. The plant climbs from 12 to 20 feet tall, vining up tall trees, which shade its growth. It is perennial, with a woody stem and ovate leaves. Small white flowers yield round berries that are red when ripe. Plants are harvested from the third to the fifteenth year of their lives.

GEOGRAPHIC LOCATION

This native of the jungles of India has been cultivated for hundreds of years and is now grown also in Malaya, Indochina, and Indonesia. In modern times the center for pepper trade is Singapore. Here, Malabar, Sumatran, and Penang pepper is wholesaled for export. Small amounts are cultivated in Madagascar and Thailand.

HISTORY

Mentioned by Roman writers in the fifth century, pepper figured in the history of Rome when Attila demanded 3,000 pounds as part of a ransom for that city.

SCENT AND APPEARANCE

The oil is liquidy, water-white to pale green-gray, but it becomes more viscous with age. The aromatic oil smells fresh, dry-woody, warm-spicy, and somewhat reminiscent of elemi. The oil is not pungent at all since these constituents do not leach out in steam distillation. There are light and heavy pepper oils: the heavy oil is most tenacious, but the light type has a very volatile top note, easily lost in improper storage.

BLENDING

Though this oil does not have wide application in regular perfumery, it can be blended with eugenol and isoeugenol for carnation and rose bases, or for oriental, amber, and dry-aldehydic bases. It is quite interesting mixed with rose. The path culminates in Netzach, which corresponds to rose, among others.

This attribution is not very satisfactory. There is more in galbanum than the Saturnian and airy elements. Galbanum is too exciting to be a truly Aquarian perfume; it is too demonic, it lacks the element of humanity.

—Aleister Crowley, 777

KEY 28 = THE STAR = GALBANUM, BERGAMOT

QABALA

Key scale #28, Trump XVII, the Star, is ruled by Aquarius; its letter is Tz; its color purple or violet; its tone A sharp. Alternatives to the unsatisfactory attribution of galbanum include spearmint, pine, and bergamot. Other possibilities include lavender oil and clary sage. This is a path of meditation and revelation. It brings insight, realization of possibilities, and hope. Other qualities include artistry, courage, creative visualization, discernment, dreaminess, faith, goal-orientation, influence over others, inspiration, intuition, peace, positive attitude, questing spirit, strength, and transcendence. In ancient times, Saturn rather than Mercury ruled this sign. Hence the Saturnian scent bergamot is ascribed, but it shares some chemistry with lavender, a Mercurial oil.

DESCRIPTION

The fresh peel of *Citrus bergamia* is distilled for the oil. The small bergamot orange grows to about 15 feet in height, but the fruits are not edible. The leaves and twigs are used to distill bergamot-petitgrain oil. Fruit is usually collected between November and February.

GEOGRAPHIC LOCATION

Bergamot is grown largely in Italy between Palmi and Brancaleone, and around the toe of the boot.

HISTORY

Roy Genders, in *Perfume Through the Ages*, (pg. 134) recounts how bergamot was produced in Lombardy from plantations of bergamot orange. It was a main ingredient in eau de cologne made of the otto of neroli, rosemary, and bergamot mixed with spirits. It was so much in demand during Napoleon's time that the supply never met the demand. Mixed with rectified spirits, extract of bergamot was widely used on handkerchiefs. In voodoo, bergamot oil is used to uncross people and protect them from misfortune and physical danger. It is also used to anoint the heads of all participants during initiation rituals.

SCENT AND APPEARANCE

The greenish otto has a smell somewhat like rosemary, but the best oil comes from the ripest fruits and is yellowish or brownish green. Bright green oil is either old or artificially tinted with copper. Fruits grown at higher altitudes yield the lightest oils, which are more rare. The top note is extremely rich and sweet-fruity; the midnote, oily-herbaceous with a balsamic dryout, somewhat reminiscent of tobacco or clary sage. Terpenes add freshness to the top note, but the terpeneless oil is a little stronger in concentration. Unlike most citrus oils, bergamot has some fixative effect (Aquarius is a fixed sign).

BLENDING

Use it for sweet freshness in citrus colognes, chypres, fougeres, and fantasy bases. Terpeneless oil is good for high-class perfumes and better florals, including lily of the valley, chypre, gardenia, lavender, and violet.

> Violet *Perfume Oil: An excellent oil for breaking the power of hexes and averting evil spells. Overcomes problems arising in marriage.*
>
> —Pelton, *The Complete Book of Voodoo*

KEY 29 = THE MOON = AMBERGRIS, VIOLET

QABALA

Key scale #29, Trump XVIII, the Moon, is Pisces and therefore lunar. Its color is magenta; letter Q; and tone B. Crowley alluded to this as a malefic path of witchcraft in its lowest sense, therefore the violet scent for warding off evil is a useful adjunct to the attribution of ambergris, which was covered extensively under Kether. This path relates to biorhythms and body consciousness, particularly that governed by the cerebellum. It is the realm of instincts and deceptions. Its feelings and qualities include bewilderment, dreaminess, empathy, fluidity, illusion, imagination, intuition, psychism, vacillation, and yearning. On this path you must face and overcome the phantoms of your own subconscious.

DESCRIPTION

Violet flower absolute comes from *Viola odorata*, which blooms from February through April. Its leaves are heart-shaped and downy (perhaps suggesting the smoothing over of tensions in love relationships). The stalks arise from a creeping rhizome. The deep purple flowers have five sepals at their base and five unequal petals. The plant propagates itself by putting out runners.

GEOGRAPHIC LOCATION

Violet is cultivated for perfume in France, Italy, China, and India. Over 200 species are widely distributed through all temperate zones and many tropical areas.

HISTORY

Violet comes from the Latin *viola*, which is derived from the Greek name *Ione*. Myth tells us that when Hera became jealous, Zeus changed his lover Io into a white heifer. Violets sprang from the earth for her food. Homer and Virgil wrote about violets. The Greeks alleged that they moderated anger. Later, the Celts used violets for cosmetics, to enhance beauty, and to combat wicked spirits. It was also prescribed for insomnia and, as this path is associated with sleep, it is germane. Napoleon used the violet as the emblem of his Imperial party.

SCENT AND APPEARANCE

Violet perfumes have ionone or methyl ionone as their base and are further modified or blended. Good synthetics contain at least some absolute. Extraction of flowers is uneconomical and so has become rare, but violet is not an especially popular scent anymore. Absolute is olive-greenish, viscous, and has a delicate, sweet-floral odor. Even before World War II, violet absolute was over $5,000 per pound.

BLENDING

Synthetic violet goes well with clove bud absolute, mimosa, boronia, ylang-ylang, sandalwood, bergamot, and other synthetics. Stellar Visions' bouquet for Quof includes anise, pine, and violet.

> Cinnamon—*the appearance is decidedly solar; any martial element therein is not confirmed by the perfume, which resembles that of a hot summer day, in the opinion of many sensitives.*
>
> —Aleister Crowley, *777*

KEY 30 = THE SUN = OLIBANUM, CINNAMON

QABALA

Key scale #30, Trump XIX, the Sun, is solar in nature; its letter is R; color yellow; and tone D natural. It represents the highest level of the human intellect, acting in accord with the body, environment, and consciousness. In some ways, this relates to a spiritualized perspective on sex. The Sun expresses brilliance, contentment, creativity, devotion, energy, enlightenment, expansion, love, playfulness, and splendor.

DESCRIPTION

Cinnamomum zeylanicum, a member of the Laurel family, likes to grow in almost pure sand. It likes constant rain and a consistently hot temperature. Trees grow from 20 to 30 feet high, but when the plants are cultivated they are pruned into large bushes. Their thick, scabrous bark is the crude material for distillation of cinnamon oil. The strong branches have speckled, greenish-orangy and leathery leaves and bear small white flowers in panicles. The fruit is an oval berry, like an acorn, which is blue with white spots with ripe. Climate and cultivation procedures affect the quality of the bark. The plant flowers in May and fruits in July. Stripped trees die, but new shoots come forth from the stump. As bark dries it rolls into quills.

GEOGRAPHIC LOCATION

Cinnamon is cultivated primarily in Ceylon, but also in Malabar (India), Cochin-China, Sumatra, Burma, Indochina, and several Indonesian islands. Cinnamon is native to east India and Indonesia. In the Seychelles, cinnamon grows wild in abundance because the talking mynah bird (*Acridotheres tristis*) loves to eat the cinnamon fruits, and so it seeds new trees constantly.

HISTORY

Before cinnamon was cultivated the Dutch held a monopoly on product harvested from the wild. Cultivation began in 1776, against Dutch opposition. They felt that cultivating the plant would destroy its value. For many years the bark was not distilled in the countries of origin. Now distillation is done in Ceylon, the Seychelles, India, and Indochina, but the oil processed in the United States and Europe is considered superior.

SCENT AND APPEARANCE

The best Ceylon bark oil is steam-distilled from the inner bark of small shoots. It is pale to dark yellow, sometimes brownish yellow. This oily liquid is extremely powerful, with a diffusive, warm-spicy, sweet, and tenacious odor. The dryness of the dry-out contrasts with the sweetness of the top note. Its main constituents, cinnamic aldehyde, eugenol, and acet-eugenol, have many specialty uses in perfume.

BLENDING

A classic base for oriental-woody notes, the warm-dry spiciness of cinnamon also goes well with olibanum. Even 1 percent of this oil in a blend gives it tremendous diffusive power, or *radiation*. High-grade oils may cost between two to two-and-one-half times as much as commercial grade, but they are definitely worth it. Since even fine oil is frequently cut with synthetic adulterants, paying a high price is no proof of receiving the finest oil. Stellar Visions' blend combines cinnamon, olibanum, and galangal for the path Resh.

> Olibanum *is the fiery elemental incense of Moses.*
>
> —Aleister Crowley, *777*

KEY 31 = JUDGEMENT/THE AEON = OLIBANUM

QABALA

Key scale #31, Trump XX, the Aeon, is ruled by the element Fire. Its color is fiery red; letter S-Sh; tone C natural. As the spirit of primal fire, this path shows the judgment the personality undergoes on its quest for inner development. A continual monitoring of progress means the dross is slowly burned away in the redeeming fire. Qualities include accomplishment, ascent, atonement, awakening, balance, decisiveness, direction, ecstasy, elation, elevation, emergence, energy, purification, realization, resurrection, revelation, and transformation.

SCENT

Olibanum is covered extensively under Tiphareth.

> *There is little difficulty in recognizing Saturnian perfumes; the difficulty in practice is to find one which is at all tolerable to the sense of smell.*
>
> —Aleister Crowley, *777*

KEY 32 = THE UNIVERSE = CYPRESS

QABALA

Key scale #32, Trump XXI, the Universe, is the last of the paths. It is the letter T-Th; the color indigo or black; and tone A natural. Incenses used for evocation on this path include asafetida, scammony, sulphur, and the like, none of which meet our purposes here. Therefore, we attribute cypress oil as a bearable alternative. This is a path of completion, concentration, crystallization, synthesis, and grounding. In its higher aspect, it is the melding of logic and intuition in perfection and attainment.

DESCRIPTION

This oil comes from the evergreen *Cypressus sempervirens*. (Do not confuse with the tropical grasses known as cyperus, which also have an oil distilled from them).

GEOGRAPHIC LOCATION

Originating in the eastern Mediterranean, this tree is cultivated in southern France, Italy, Corsica, Sardinia, north Africa, Spain, Portugal, and the Balkans.

HISTORY

Most distillation of this oil happens during annual pruning of these trees, which are used as windbreaks. Thus limited quantities are available for limited times. Sometimes other varieties of cypress are inadvertently mixed in, so oil lots can vary. So-called cypress oil from areas other than the Mediterranean is actually from different species. Despite its scarcity, the price of this oil is comparable to good pine needle oil. Cypress oil is used in voodoo to attract good luck, to bring financial gain, and to heal.

SCENT AND APPEARANCE

True cypress oil is pale yellow to olive-greenish with a fresh balsamic odor, like pine needles. Poucher claims that, on evaporation, it resembles ambergris. Others, too, compare the dryout to amber and labdanum-amber. Partially deterpenized oil is best for blending with cistus oil.

BLENDING

Stellar Visions' blend for Tav includes cypress, myrrh, and civet, all Saturnian scents. Cypress oil also goes well with cistus oil, lavender oil, mandarin oil, clary sage, musk ambrette or macrocyclic musks, storax, and chamomile oil.

Aeone, Nymph of Venus

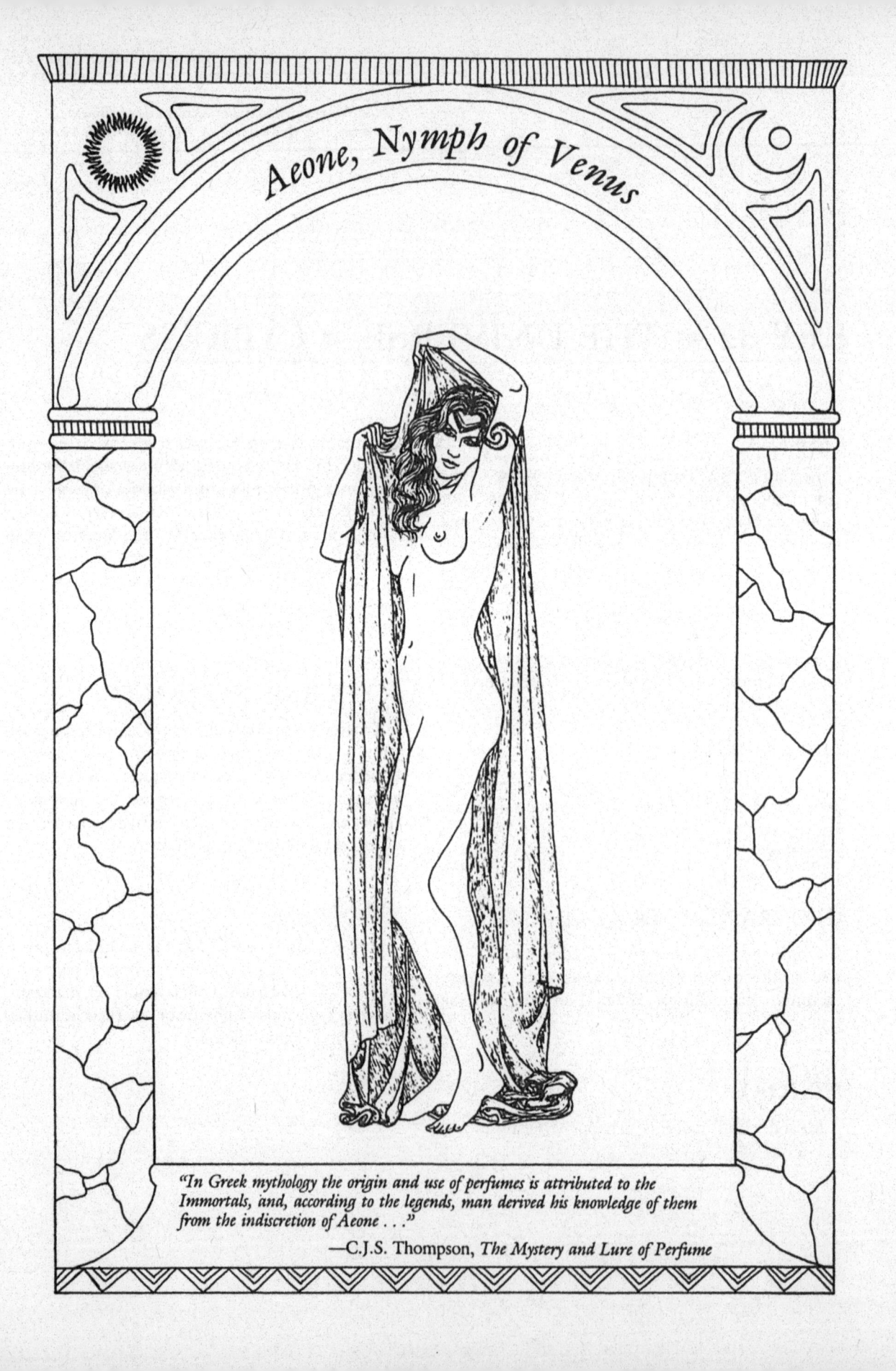

"In Greek mythology the origin and use of perfumes is attributed to the Immortals, and, according to the legends, man derived his knowledge of them from the indiscretion of Aeone..."

—C.J.S. Thompson, *The Mystery and Lure of Perfume*

Chapter 7

PLANETARY PERFUMES AND THEIR GOD-FORMS

Ceremonies, vestments, perfumes, characters and figures being, as we have stated, necessary to apply imagination to the education of the will, the success of magical work depends upon the faithful observation of all the Rites, which are in no sense fantastic or arbitrary. They have been transmitted to us by antiquity or obtained permanently by the essential laws of analogical realization and of the correspondence which interbinds ideas and forms.

—Eliphas Levi, *Transcendental Magic*, 249

Astrological attributions of scents are of three types: (1) scents that correspond to the four elements, (2) fragrances that correspond to the planets; and (3) scents that share harmonies with the signs of the zodiac. We have already seen how some scents relate to planets and signs in the zodiac through the Qabala, but there are many others besides the primary ones. There are also many ways to use them, ranging from very simple to highly complex.

The simplest daily ritual requires standing before a full-length mirror and contemplating the fullness of your being. Anoint yourself with your ritual oil, take three deep breaths (breathe in, "I am"; breathe out, "At ease"), then close your eyes. In your mind's eye, picture yourself as you would like to be—your master-self. See the colors and shapes, hear the sounds, and feel the feelings of that higher you, as you inhale your fragrance of choice. Spend several minutes imagining your face, your gestures, your actions, and your interrelationships with others. Finally, after this affirmation of your highest ideal, open your eyes and start your day.

THE FOUR ELEMENTS

The simplest division of the signs of the Zodiac is into the four elements of fire, water, air, and earth. Each sign is assigned as follows:

Fire: Aries, Leo, Sagittarius
Water: Cancer, Scorpio, Pisces
Air: Gemini, Libra, Aquarius
Earth: Taurus, Virgo, Capricorn

This division reflects the division of the circle, as a symbol of wholeness, into four quadrants. The fourfold division is an expression of the potential characteristics of balance, solidity, and regularity. Western civilization generally distinguishes four seasons, four directions, and four quarters of the heavens. Ritually, the sacred aspect of this quadrature is enacted in the banishing ritual and other models for the re-creation of the Universe (see Mircea Eliade's *The Sacred and the Profane* for details). Ritually placing oneself in a quadrated circle is equivalent to orienting yourself at the sacred center of the universe. In effect, you make yourself the center of the universe—your own universe, at least.

Since this quaternary system of orientation is so basic, it is not surprising that the early Greek philosophers came to the conclusion that all things are made through the combination of these four fundamental materials. Historically, as the views on matter became more refined in the West, various physical interpretations have been assigned to these symbolic elements, but their symbolic qualities remain constant.

Fire	Nitrogen	Electricity	"Strong force"
Water	Hydrogen	Liquids	"Weak force"
Air	Oxygen	Gases	Electromagnetism
Earth	Carbon	Solids	Gravity

Fire and air are thought to express masculine qualities. They are active, positive, and creative. Water and earth, seen as being feminine in nature, are passive, negative, and receptive, or yielding. Fire is known as the spiritual element and is associated with aspiration, energy, purification, and transformation. Water is the universal medium, the unfathomable depths of the human subconscious. Air is associated with breath, soul, and flights of the imagination. Earth expresses solidity and practicality, as well as the physical body. The ideal, or perfected, person is a combination of these forces.

The four elements relate directly to the most basic practice of circle magic. This type of ritual is a good place to start incorporating the use of magical oil blends. Each of the quadrants, or directions of the compass, is assigned a scent and a visualization. Stellar Visions, a supplier of the purest magical oils, uses these combinations for the elements:

Fire (direction, south)—coriander, basil, cinnamon, olibanum

Water (direction, west)—jasmine, lemon, birch, nard

Air (direction, east)—galbanum, fennel, lavender, mastic

Earth (direction, north)—vetiver, verbena, dill, rose

Because of the interaction of scent and memory, if you use these scents in the banishing ritual and concentrate on the images, you will anchor your very best visualizations to these scents. The images and feelings will be encoded holistically in your memory for future automatic retrieval. Concentration can then give way to greater spontaneity.

Another application of these scents to the four elements is a short series of meditations for balancing one's energies. When matter is conceived as consisting of four divisions, the psyche is also perceived that way. In magic, this fourfold division is expressed as the four powers of the Sphinx. The Sphinx is a mythological creature whose androgynous nature combines both masculine and feminine elements. It represents the real Self, which has the answers to the riddle of existence and the universe.

In the four powers of the Sphinx meditation, the aspirant seeks an equilibrated development of the forces of nature. This balanced strength is expressed in the axiom, "To Will, to Dare, to Know, to Keep Silent." These four powers correspond to the fixed signs of the zodiac to represent the elements. Use the oil of each element for a meditation period on its qualities.

The following symbols, corresponded by Crowley, may be used as the basis for the meditation:

The Four Powers of the Sphinx

	MOTTO	SIGN	SYMBOL	ATTRIBUTES
Fire	To Dare	Leo	Lion	Strength, courage
Water	To Keep Silent	Scorpio	Man	Sublety, spiritual wisdom
Air	To Know	Aquarius	Eagle	Swift, soaring intelligence
Earth	To Will	Taurus	Bull	Patience, solid energy

Begin your guided visualization by closing your eyes and taking three deep breaths, slowly inhaling the essence of Earth. Picture the astrological symbol of Taurus in vibrant, glowing color, perhaps on a shimmering curtain or floating in a mist. Next, step through the curtain or mist to a scene that depicts all the salient features of the earth element as you know it. Explore this region fully for colors, plants, animals, whatever you can find that has meaning for you. Traveling, in imagination, to the center of this region, encounter the bull as the central symbol of this domain. Look at it, feel empathy with it, then merge with its consciousness. Contemplate the qualities of groundedness, patience, and solid energy. When finished, let that scene dissolve and imagine returning to your point of origin, and step back through the veil to "normal" awareness. Record your experience in a journal.

Journey in the same manner to the realms of fire, air, and water. Although it could be done in one sitting, it is probably best to do the meditation over five nights, one for each element and the final one for their synthesis. This way, each scent will be experienced in isolation, providing an uncontaminated memory, and the effects of your meditations will have time to establish themselves in your personality. Combining the olfactory input of the perfumes with visualizations and other sense-based inputs is a surefire way of acquiring new resources.

Finish your meditation on the elements by visualizing them unified in the image of the Sphinx. Step into the image and identify with it. What do you see, hear, feel, and experience as the Sphinx? Its wings correspond to air, female breasts to water, bull's body to earth, and lion's claws to fire. To paraphrase the French magician, Levi, TO DARE we must KNOW; TO WILL, we must DARE; We must WILL to possess empire; and to reign we must BE SILENT.

PLANETARY PERFUMES

As Crowley pointed out, "At one time or another mediaeval writers on magic have attributed every possible incense to every possible planet." The contradictions in tradition, combined with the wide variety in individual perception, make any concise spiritual attribution illusive. The only answer, therefore, is to experiment for yourself to understand the virtues of the perfumes. They are important since, according to Crowley, "they constitute the most vital link between the material and astral planes...." Gentle heating of the oil, either on the body or in a small ceramic dish with a candle under it, is all that is necessary to activate the volatile oils. They should never be burned.

The famous French magician Eliphas Levi offered some corresponding perfumes for the days of the week, with appropriate ritual forms for their employment. These attributions are harmonious, if not identical with Crowley's. This seems reasonable and likely, since Crowley claims to have been this famous magician in one of his past lives! He sets forth the planetary rites in *Transcendental Magic* as follows:

> Magical works are also seven in number: (1) works of light and riches, under the auspices of the Sun; (2) works of divination and mystery, under the invocation of the Moon; (3) works of skill, science and eloquence, under the protection of Mercury; (4) works of wrath and chastisement, consecrated to Mars; (5) works of love, favored by Venus; (6) works of ambition and intrigue, under the influence of Jupiter; (7) works of malediction and death, under the patronage of Saturn.

In order of the days of the week, Eliphas Levi's preparations for the rites follow.

SUN —The Magus who intends to undertake the works of light must operate on a *Sunday*, from midnight to eight in the morning, or from three in the afternoon to ten in the evening. He should wear a purple vestment, with tiara and vestments of gold. The altar of perfumes and the tripod of sacred fire must be encircled by wreaths of laurel, heliotrope and sunflowers; the perfumes are *cinnamon*, strong incense [*frankincense*], *saffron* and *red sandal*; the ring must be of gold, with a chrysolith or ruby; the carpet must be of lion-skins, the fans of sparrow-hawk feathers.

☽ **MOON** —On *Monday* the robe is white, embroidered with silver, and having a triple collar of pearls, crystals and selenite; the tiara must be covered with yellow silk, emblazoned with silver characters forming the Hebrew monogram of Gabriel, as given in the *Occult Philosophy* of Agrippa; the perfumes are *white sandal, camphor, amber, aloes* and pulverized seeds of cucumber; the wreaths are mugwort, moonwort, and yellow ranunculuses. Tapestries, garments and objects of a black color must be avoided; and no metal except silver should be worn on the person.

♂ **MARS** —On *Tuesday*, a day for the operations of vengeance, the color of the vestment should be that of flame, rust, or blood, with belt and bracelets of steel. The tiara must be bound with gold; the wand must not be used, but only the magical dagger and sword; the wreaths must be of absinth and rue, the ring of steel, with an amethyst for precious stone.

☿ **MERCURY** —On *Wednesday*, a day favorable for transcendent science, the vestment should be green, or shot with various colors; the necklace of pearls in hollow glass beads containing mercury; the perfumes *benzoin, mace* and *storax*; the flowers narcissus, lily, herb-mercury, fumitory and marjoram; the jewel should be the agate.

♃ **JUPITER** —On *Thursday*, a day of great religious and political operations, the vestment should be scarlet and on the forehead should be worn a brass tablet, with the character of the spirit of Jupiter, and the three words: GIARAR, BETHOR, SAMGABIEL; the perfumes are incense, *ambergris, balm, grain of paradise; macis* and *saffron*; the ring must be enriched with an emerald or sapphire; the wreaths and crowns should be oak, poplar, fig and pomegranate leaves.

♀ **VENUS** —On *Friday*, the day for amorous operations, the vestment should be of sky-blue, the hangings of green and rose, the ornaments of polished copper, the crowns of violets, the wreaths of *roses*, myrtle and olive; the ring should be enriched with a turquoise; lapis-lazuli and beryl will answer for tiara and clasps; the fans must be of swan's feathers;

TABLE 6 Conway's Planetary Correspondences

PLANET	COLOR	PLANT	METAL	GEM	PERFUMES
Sun	Orange	Sunflower, heliotrope, chicory	Gold	Topaz, diamond	Aloe wood, saffron, cloves, cinnamon, myrrh
Moon	Violet	Hazel, almond, peony	Silver	Crystal, pearl, quartz	Camphor, jasmine, frankincense, white sandalwood
Mercury	Yellow	Vervain, palm, cinquefoil	Quicksilver	Agate, opal	Cinnamon, mace, cloves, narcissus, storax
Venus	Emerald green	Rose, myrtle, fennel, vervain, maidenhair	Copper	Emerald, turquoise	Ambergris, sandalwood, musk, benzoin, pink rose, myrtle
Mars	Scarlet	Absinth, rue, lambstongue	Iron	Ruby	Benzoin, sulphur, tobacco
Jupiter	Blue	Narcissus, oak, poplar, agrimony	Tin	Amethyst, sapphire	Nutmeg, cinnamon, balm, cloves, aloes wood
Saturn	Indigo	Ash, yew, cypress, houseleek	Lead	Onyx, sapphire	Civet, musk, alum

and the operator must wear upon his breast a copper talisman with the character of Anael and the words: AVEEVA, VADELILITH.

♄ *SATURN* —On *Saturday*, a day of funereal operations, the vestment must be black or brown, with characters embroidered in orange or black silk; round the neck must be worn a lamina of lead, with the character of Saturn and the words: ALMALEC, APHIEL, ZARAHIEL; the perfumes should be *diagridrium, scammony, alum, sulphur* and *assafoetida*; the ring should be adorned with an onyx; the garlands should be of ash, cypress and hellebore; on the onyx of the ring, during the hours of Saturn, the double head of Janus should be engraved with the consecrated awl.

David Conway, in *Magic: An Occult Primer*, gives a very similar list with different correspondences in tabular form (see Table 6). His table includes "the physical details which you will bring into your ritual so as to link your subconscious with the astral world." Since these attributions differ from Levi's our best recommendation is that you experiment with them yourself and evaluate your results.

The principal use of the perfumes is psychological. The whole apparatus of the correspondences—weapons, colors, symbols, and scents—help to intoxicate the senses. The choice of substances and symbolism, in fact, determines the nature of the ceremony. The perfume brings with it the atmosphere of the appropriate planetary influence into the operation. There is an old alchemical notion that when a substance is burned, its vapors represent its "spirit."

ZODIAC SCENTS

Yet another series of attributions for scents and the signs of the zodiac is provided by the modern witch, Sybil Leek, in *Sybil Leek's Astrological Guide to Successful Everyday Living*. Her attributions are as follows:

♈ ***ARIES*** —Your nose is highly alerted to smell. Such things as cedarwood chests and odoriferous woods such as pine and cypress appeal to you. Flower perfume—attar of roses.

TABLE 7 Planetary Perfumes

	ZODIACAL BLENDS
♈	coriander, pine, basil, cinnamon, tarragon, cardamom
♉	geranium, dill, jasmine, myrtle, patchouli, vanilla
♊	anise, lavender, mace, basil, mastic, bay
♋	jasmine, aloe, lemon, lavender, orris, nard
♌	cinnamon, myrrh, nutmeg, ambergris, olibanum, allspice
♍	mastic, olibanum, lavender, spearmint, fennel, bergamot
♎	rose, birch, galbanum, cypress, spearmint, cedar
♏	musk, pine, allspice, galangal, ginger, violet
♐	hyssop, dill, clove, aloe, cedar, pine
♑	cedar, vetiver, wormwood, myrrh, bay, cypress
♒	myrrh, spearmint, pine, bergamot, cypress, eucalyptus
♓	violet, patchouli, nutmeg, cedar, anise, pine
	PLANETARY BLENDS
♄	civet, myrrh, patchouli, cypress, vetiver
♃	cedar, nutmeg, anise, hyssop, clove
♂	pine, basil, allspice, musk, coriander
♀	rose, violet, vanilla, civet, ylang-ylang
☿	mastic, fennel, dill, lavender, calamus
☽	orris, camphor, jasmine, lemon, birch
☉	cinnamon, galangal, ambergris, bay, olibanum
	ELEMENTAL BLENDS
🜂	coriander, basil, cinnamon, olibanum
🜄	jasmine, birch, myrrh, nard
🜁	galbanum, fennel, lavender, mastic
🜃	vetiver, verbena, dill, rose

- ♉ **TAURUS** —Musk, rose, carnation, honeysuckle, violet, saffron, and satinwood.

- ♊ **GEMINI** —Fresh sparkling colognes from a fresh flower base, in preference to heady perfume essences. Bayberry, mastic resin, sandalwood.

- ♋ **CANCER** —You enjoy all fragrant leaves, all odorous vegetables, and most forms of tree and plant life, such as : aloe, bay leaves, camphor, cedar, myrtle, cinnamon, sandalwood, poppy.

- ♌ **LEO** —Red sandalwood, frankincense, camphor, cassia, clove.

- ♍ **VIRGO** —All woodland and fruit perfumes rather than sweet, flowery ones: bayberry, cinnamon, citron peel, red and yellow sander, mace, mystic resin.

- ♎ **LIBRA** —Jasmine; musk; rose; violet; all mild perfumes, preferably from a flower base; satinwood and sandalwood.

- ♏ **SCORPIO** —All fragrances from odoriferous woods, pine, yucca, rosemary, cypress, briar roses, dogwood.

- ♐ **SAGITTARIUS** —All odoriferous fruits; nutmeg; saffron; clove.

- ♑ **CAPRICORN** —Fragrance from all odoriferous roots; frankincense; khus khus.

- ♒ **AQUARIUS** —All odoriferous roots, frankincense, pine, pepperwort.

- ♓ **PISCES** —Clove, nutmeg, fragrance from all odoriferous fruits or exotic tropical flowers such as those found in Hawaii.

SCENTS AND ASSUMING THE GOD-FORM:

A more complex method of utilizing planetary scents is with the ritual known as the assumption of god-forms. To perform this rite, the aspirant first creates the sacred circle as a working area. The modern magician then proceeds to create a vivid picture of a deity's characteristic appearance, attributes, symbols, and myths. This image is built in the mind, detail by detail, and is concentrated on while the god is invoked. Once again, the perfumes form an integral part of this image-building process.

Once the picture is crystal clear in the mind's eye, the magician identifies with what he or she has pictured. These god-forms represent great universal forces or currents, or aspects of cosmic life, but they also exist in the human mind. The great twentieth-century psychologist, Carl Jung, spoke of them as archetypes and reiterated their importance in the process of human development and maturation.

Jung said that forms or images of a collective nature occur practically all over the earth and are expressed in myths and folklore. These archetypes well up from our subconscious as "fundamental patterns of symbol formation." The importance is not found in the actual symbol but in the possibility of connection to the deeper mind that it makes possible. Connecting with these powerful symbols helps us feel more whole and connected to the sacred source of life.

Invoking these god-forms through ritual is done through mimesis or imitation of the qualities of life events of these mythical figures. The ritual is the external form of an internal union or state of grace. It helps us break the barriers of the ego to experience something greater than ourselves. Once again, scents can be used to anchor these positive, connecting experiences.

The God-Forms

Apollo/The Sun

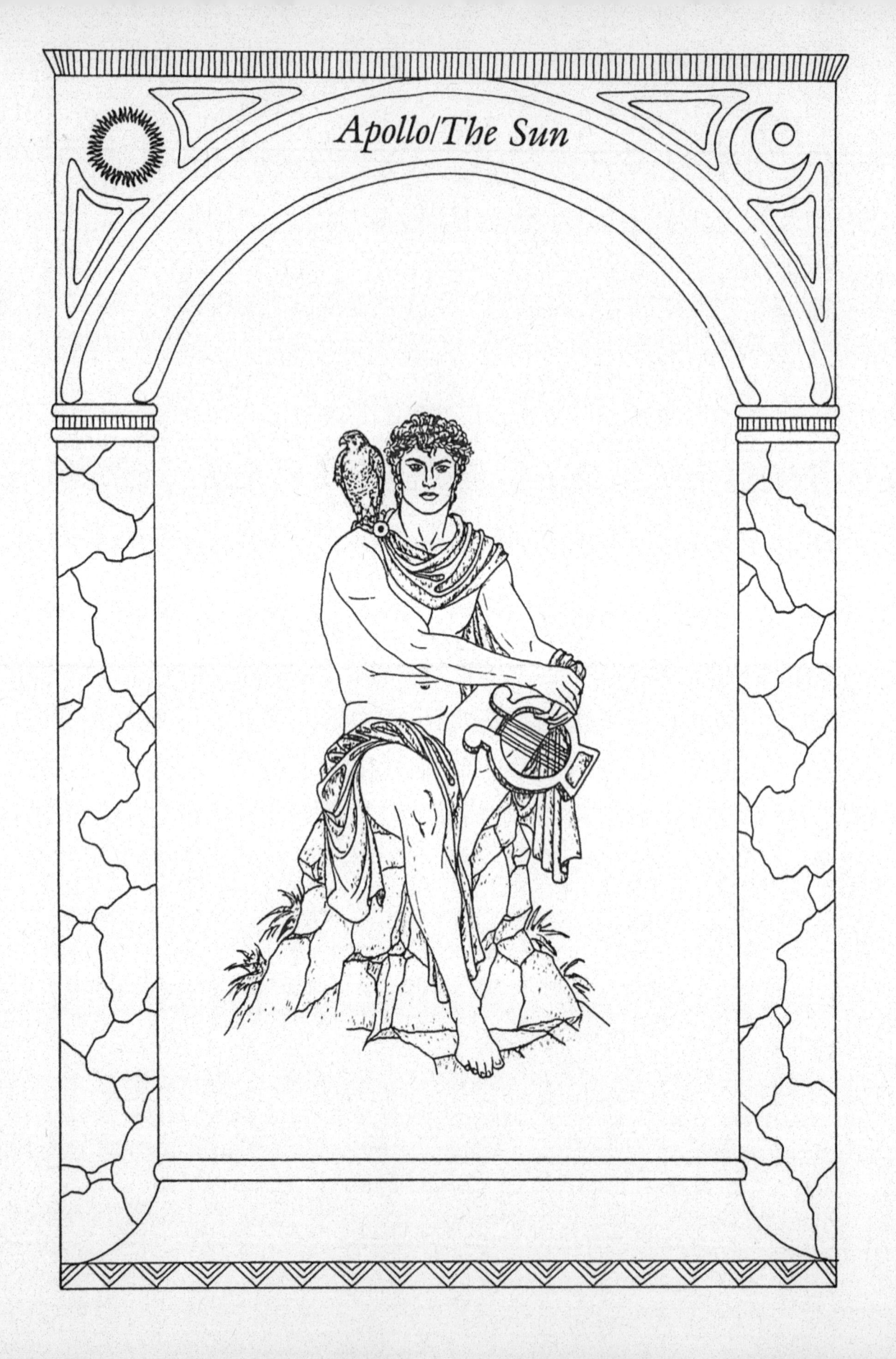

A Greek inscription on the ruins of the temple of Apollo at Miletus records the gifts made to the shrine of Seleceucus II, King of Syria (246–227 B.C.) which consisted of two vessels of gold and silver, ten talents of frankincense, and one of myrrh.

THE SUN = APOLLO

ASTROLOGICAL SYMBOLISM

The Sun is regarded as representing the center of the field of consciousness—the ego. This contrasts somewhat with Qabala, where the sun represents the self, or higher mind. But in both cases the sun has an integrating function in the psyche. The sign and house our natal sun is in tells us how we try to achieve our goals and develop in accordance with our innermost desires. To paraphrase John Sanford in *Dreams and Healing*, the sun as a symbol often appears in religious lore as a symbol for God; Christ is often represented as the rising sun. The Aztecs regarded Huitzilopochtli, seen as identical with the sun, as the god on whom all human welfare depended. To American Indians, the sun is a symbol of the Great Spirit and the object of prayer and reverence.

The sun is also a symbol for the archetype of masculine consciousness, just as the moon is feminine. It is thought that the *yang* power sees everything in the startlingly clear light of the sun as *yin* sees it by the shimmering moonlight, which fuses things together even as sunlight differentiates things. Dreams emphasizing the sun or rising sun show that this archetype of wholeness is assuming more importance in your life. Keywords include ambition, artistry, creativity, dynamism, energy, enlightenment, healing, inspiration, intelligence, leadership, music, organization, self-confidence, spirituality, vitality, warmth, and will power.

GOD-FORM VISUALIZATION

Solar gods from the cultures of the world are Apollo, Ra, Osiris, Mithras, Christ, and Krishna, among others. Though some magical orders have employed Egyptian god-forms for their rites, modern Jungian psychologists usually speak of archetypal powers in the more human Greek forms. Therefore, we offer a visualization of Apollo:

Crowned with laurel leaves, a young man of idealized beauty lounges on a sun-drenched mountain peak as he relaxes after the hunt. His broad chest and slim hips adorn his vigorous body. He is beardless, but his high forehead is crowned by ringlets of thick golden hair, which is knotted at the nape of his neck. He relaxes nude in the summer air with his flowing cape thrown casually across a shoulder. His bow and quiver await nearby, while he picks up his lyre to offer a haunting melody. Farther down the mountain, in his temple of healing, divination and prophecy are practiced. His sacred animals abound in the area: swan, cock, crow, lion, vulture, hawk, wolf, and serpent. Laurels, palms, olives, and tamarisk mingle in his garden with marigold, heliotrope, sunflowers, eucalyptus, and acacia, but the fragrant frankincense pervades his temples. He is the light which ripens the fruit, both agricultural and human. His familiars are the muses, patrons of the arts and sciences, who wander through the garden.

Approach the celestial radiance of Apollo with *clear consciousness*.

PLANETARY OILS

Master perfumer Lady Sara Cunningham-Carter attributes the following astral scents to the Sun in *The Arts Magian*.

ACACIA OIL (Robinia Pseudacacia)—Used to purify the altar and anoint ritual equipment, and to aid in psychic development and meditation.

ANGELICA OIL (Archangelica officinalis)—Used for spiritual power, protection, magical energy, and in evocational rituals. Root oil is preferred to seed oil. Blend with patchouli, opoponax, clary sage, oakmoss, and coumarin for chypres and oriental bases, or in cologne. This oil is extremely strong; use it sparingly. Base note.

AZALEA OIL (Azalea pontica)—Used to promote success and advancement in your career.

BAY OIL (Myria acris)—Used to counteract negativity, ward off evil, and stimulate psychic vision. This leaf oil blends with lavender, citrus, rosemary, geraniol, cinnamic alcohol, and ylang-ylang. Top note.

CHAMOMILE OIL (Matricaria chamomilla)—Used for blessing, increasing finances, and as an anointing oil in healings. The German, Hungarian, or "blue" oils are the best for a warm, rich undertone in citrus colognes, amber-, chypre-, and fougere-bases, and with lavender and pine. Top note.

CASSIA OIL (Cinnamomum cassia)—Worn to attract wealth, happiness, success and to promote one's station in life. With its cinnamic undertone it is used with ionones, bergamot, orris, olibanum, and ylang-ylang. Middle note.

CINNAMON OIL (cinnamomum zeylanicum)—Worn to attract good fortune, anoint the head, and bless rooms. Middle note.

CLOVE OIL (Eugenia caryophyllata)—Worn as an aphrodisiac oil of attraction, it is also used as an energy booster in solar perfumes and incenses. Clove bud, leaf, and stem oil are all different: bud oil is best with vanilla, rose, honeysuckle, lavender, clary sage, bergamot, bay, and ylang-ylang. Middle note.

EUCALYPTUS OIL (Eucalyptus globulus)—Used in healing wounds and worn for protection from evil and mental anguish. Use with rosemary, lavender, thyme, and Spanish sage. Top note.

FRANKINCENSE OIL (Juniperus lycia)—Used for blessing, protection, cleansing, consecration, and to attract success and prosperity. Base note.

GALANGAL OIL (Alpinia officinarum)—Used to attract success and prosperity, and to avoid legal problems. It is also used in blends for healing. Blend with lavender, pine, citrus, rosemary, patchouli, myrtle, and opoponax.

GRAINS OF PARADISE OIL (Amomum melegueta)—Used to attract success in one's desires, it is used in "love" blends as a sexual stimulant. It has a peppery odor.

HELIOTROPE OIL (Heliotropium grandiflorum)—Used as an aid in prayer, meditation, and psychic and spiritual development, it is also used to restore peace and harmony and aid in spirit communication. It is not commercially available.

LEMON-GRASS OIL (Cymbopogon citratus)—Opens the psychic centers and aids one in spirit communication. Ionones are processed out of this oil.

LINALOOL OIL (Copal limon)—Used as an anointing oil in healing, it is very soothing and calming to the nerves. Both seed and wood oils are available, but wood oil is preferred for delicate blends like muguet, lilac, apple blossom, freesia, rose, and sweet pea. Top note.

MARIGOLD OIL (Tagetes patula)—Used to attract success and prosperity. Blends with oakmoss and tea-leaf extract. Has a dark, intense color. Top note.

PASSIONFLOWER OIL (Passiflor alata)—Used for blessing, for anointing ritual or devotional objects, to promote affection, and as an aid in prayer. Not commercially available.

PEONY OIL (*Paeonia montana*)—Aids in psychic development and is often used as an aid in meditation; used to encourage prophetic dreaming when applied prior to retiring.

PETITGRAIN CITRONNIER OIL (*Citrus medica*)—Used as an aid in healing. Can replace neroli in citrus colognes and blends with lavender, sage, rosemary, and olibanum. Top note.

ROSEMARY OIL (*Rosmarinus officinalis*)—Used as protection against black magic, it is also calming and healing. Lots vary markedly; blend with citrus cologne, olibanum and spice oils, lavender, origanum, pine, labdanum, olibanum, cedar, petitgrain, and nitro musks. Stops hatred and overcomes fear; for ritual bath.

SAFFRON OIL (*Crocus sativus*)—Used as a personal anointing oil to aid and develop clairvoyance. Not commercially available.

Artemis/The Moon

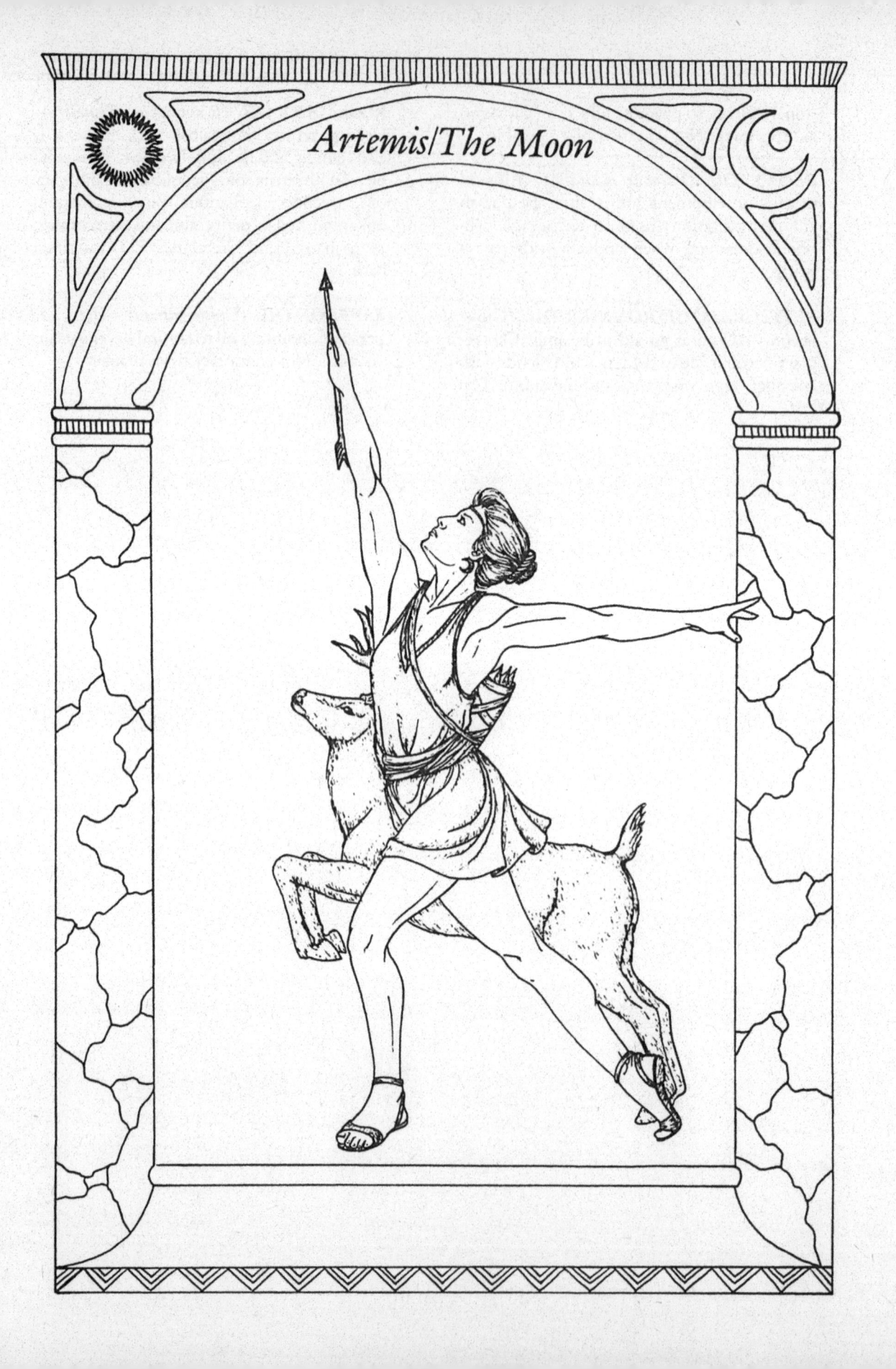

O Diana, sweet goddess, I know that thou art near me, for I have recognized thy balmy odour.

—Euripides, *Phaedra*

THE MOON = ARTEMIS

ASTROLOGICAL SYMBOLISM

The Moon represents the quality of reflectiveness. In general the moon represents the unconscious, but it also reveals the subliminal patterns of our emotional lives. The moon also relates to the archetypal feminine and therefore to cycles of life, death, and reproduction. Our conscious habit patterns can be changed by increasing awareness and reprogramming. Imagination is a valuable tool for this and guides us through the realm of the psyche, with its symbols, myths, and legends. On the deep level of unconscious life we encounter the feminine rituals that concern virginity, androgyny, initiation, and childbearing.

Keywords include adaptability, anima, containment, contemplation, cycles, divination, emotionalism, feelings, flexibility, form-giving creativity, imagination, interiority, intuition, multinatured, mothering, mystical, nourishing, nurturing, passivity, piety, protection, purity, psychic, receptivity, reflection, soulfulness, subliminal, support, sympathy, and yin energy.

GOD-FORM VISUALIZATION

Lunar goddesses are as numerous as those for the sun. Some of them include the Great Mother, the White Goddess, the Madonna, Isis, Diana, Artemis, Selene, Hekate, Kwan Yin, and all virgin goddesses. Jung called the moon the "sister and bride, mother and spouse of the sun." He also reminded us of the importance of recognizing this goddess when he declared, "Anyone who seeks to unite the opposites [conscious and unconscious] certainly needs Diana to be propitious to him." There are three major aspects of the moon: the youthful virgin, the mature, motherly woman, the mystical wise woman, who is whole within herself, or once again "virgin." Artemis embodies these in a timeless eternity.

As we invoke Artemis in our imagination, we first see her deep in the woods with her brother Apollo. They are accompanied by their retinue of heroes, centaurs, hunting dogs, and falcons. We see they are clad in hunting gear with no frivolous finery except for their matching turquoise rings. Night after night they have roamed through the deep forest seeking the deer. The young virgin is slim and supple with narrow hips and an athletic body, which gives her an androgynous quality. She has regular features, but her beauty is a little severe and she knots her hair back tightly. She wears a short tunic, tucked into her girdle to maximize her mobility. She is agile as a gazelle, fluid as molten silver. Stopping to rest, she suddenly changes before our eyes into an older woman lost in mystic contemplation. We smell the mingling of jasmine, gardenia, violet, and lotus flowers. As she gazes at us serenely, we intuitively know that she is a trusted guide to the innermost realms of the soul. We feel nourished and nurtured by her mere presence. Dim moonlight illuminates her nearby temple. We see that it is composed of brilliant crystal, studded with pearls and moonstones.

Approach her with *equanimity* and *piety*, or *purity of heart*.

PLANETARY OILS

Lady Sara's attributions for the Moon include the following:

ALOE VERA OIL (*Aloe vulgaris*)—Used in healings for its calming effect, it is also used as a psychic stimulator. Nurturing, healing aspect of the moon.

AMARYLLIS OIL (*Amarylis belladonna*)—Calming and soothing, it is also used as an aid to induce prophetic dreaming.

CAMPHOR OIL (*Cinnamomum camphora*)—Used as a psychic energizer and occult power source in lunar blends, it is also a body rub for strength.

CELERY SEED OIL (*Apium graveolens*)—Mentally cleansing and clearing, it is often used in psychic workings and by people who need to channel their thoughts. Use small amounts in florals, orientals, and lavender. Middle note.

CUCUMBER OIL (*Cucumis sativus*)—Very healing vibrations, it soothes and clears the mind.

ELECAMPANE OIL (*Inula helenium*)—Used as an aid in psychic development and meditation. Use in heavy-woody, oriental, and amber bases. Blend with cananga, cinnamon, labdanum, lavender, mimosa, olibanum, orris, tuberose, violet, cedarwood, patchouli, and nitro musks.

FRANGIPANI OIL (*Plumieria rubra*)—Excellent oil for psychic work, it also helps restore peace and harmony with its soothing vibrations. Most so-called frangipani is a synthesized fantasy perfume. The rare oil blends into honeysuckle, gardenia, tuberose, lilac, and muguet.

GARDENIA OIL (*Gardenia florida*)—Protective, calming, and soothing, it is used to heal quarrels and restore peace and love in marriage. Synthetics have replaced the floral absolute, which was used for an intense, sweet-green floral note.

GINSENG OIL (*Panax schinseng*)—Worn for physical vitality and auric healing; not readily available; English Leather makes a ginseng cologne.

JASMINE OIL (*Jasminium grandiflorum*)—Worn for blessings, protection, and good luck. Also used as a devotional anointing oil. Middle note. Cool smelling.

JUNIPER OIL (*Juniperus communis*)—Used for meditation and as an aid in gaining spiritual enlightenment due to its psychic stimulation. Blend with labdanum, mastic, opoponax, fir, oakmoss, elemi, cypress, clary sage, lovage, and benzoin.

LOTUS OIL (*Nymphea alba, Nymphea lotus*)—Used for healing, energy, and fertility; it is also said to attract good fortune and love while promoting long life.

MIMOSA OIL (*Acacia dealbata, A. floribunda*)—Used as an aid in prophetic dreaming, it is also used in healing for its calming and soothing vibrations. Blend with ionones, isoeugenol, lavandin, ylang-ylang, cinnamic alcohol, storax, and linalool.

STEPHANOTIS OIL (*Stephanotis floribunda*)—Lends personal magnetism as a sensual oil of attraction.

SWEET PEA OIL (*Lathyrus odoratus*)—Used to promote friendships and attract a lover; bouqueted from tuberose, orange flower, jasmine, rose de mai, vanilla, petitgrain, storax, benzoin, tolu, cinnamic alcohol, and other synthetics.

TUBEROSE OIL (*Polianthes tuberose*)—Used to ward off evil and negativity, it restores happiness, peace, and harmony. Although it calms the nerves it is also used as a psychic stimulator. Very expensive, it is used for frangipani, stephanotis, lilac, heliotrope, gardenia, violet, and opoponax blends. Middle note.

WALLFLOWER OIL (*Cheiranthus cheiri*)—
Used to promote peace and harmony, it is also worn to attract the assistance of good spirits. If you can get any, it blends with jasmine, ylang-ylang, tuberose, petitgrain, linalool, neroli, and isoeugenol.

Hermes/Mercury

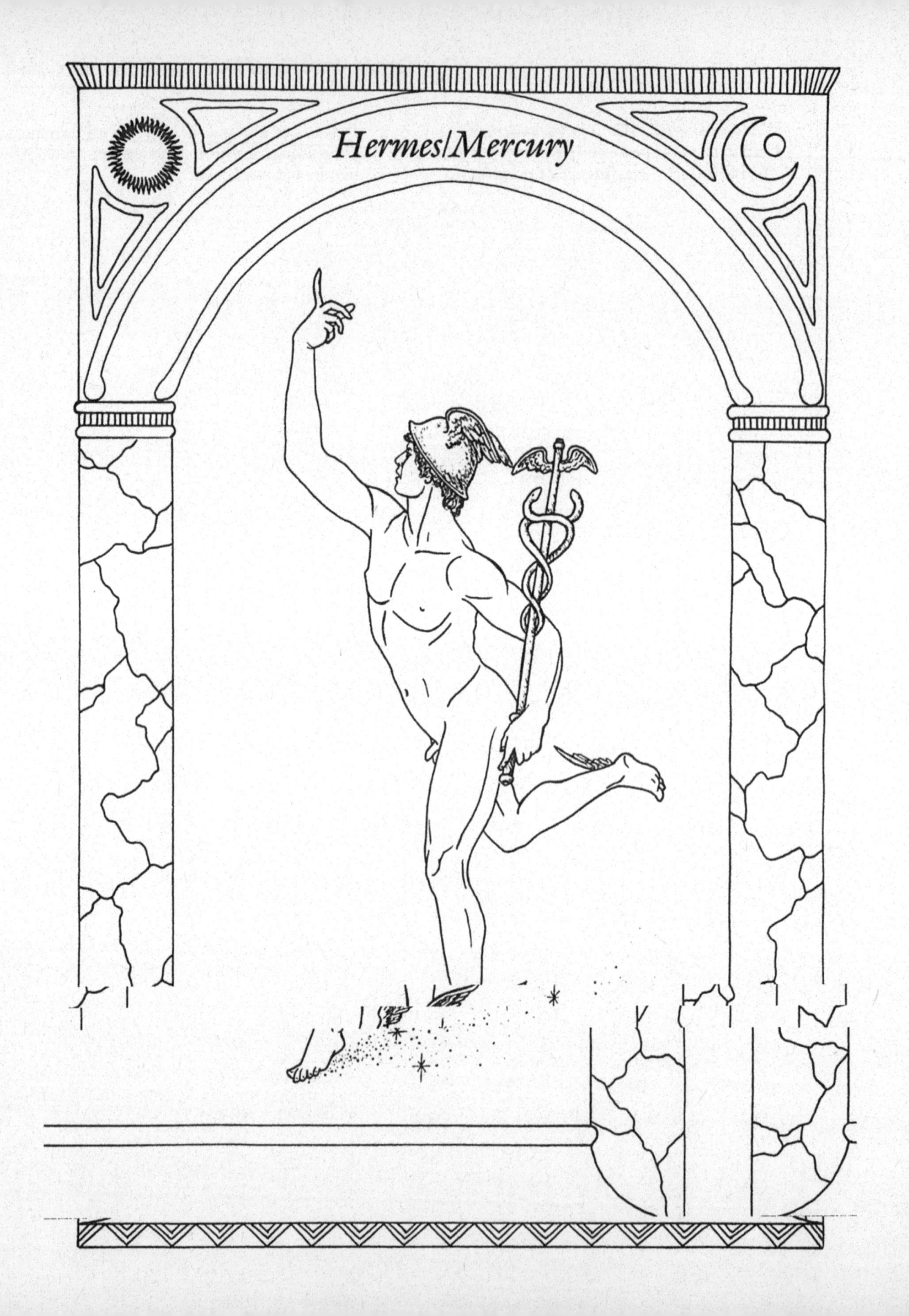

> ... *a marvelous fragrance wafted around the holy mountain and many tender-footed sheep pastured up there.*
>
> —"The Hymn to Hermes," *The Homeric Hymns*, trans. Charles Boer

MERCURY = HERMES

ASTROLOGICAL SYMBOLISM

Mercury in your chart expresses your mental abilities, ability to assimilate experiences and factual data, and communication skills. It stimulates our innate drive to classify, study, and analyze our experiences and nature. It also means becoming aware of our unconscious motivations and assimilating them through meditation and analysis. Mercury helps us see deeply into ourselves and others.

Keywords include adaptability, analysis, classification, contemplation, cunning, dexterity, eloquence, exchanging, facility, good luck, humor, intellectual curiosity, interpretation, perspective, quick-wittedness, rationality, relatedness, restlessness, self-expression, shamanism, skillfulness, trickster, writing talent.

GOD-FORM VISUALIZATION

Mercury, or Hermes, is the archetypal Trickster or magician. Hermes was the guide to the underworld of the psyche and the original boundary-breaker. He carried messages from gods to men and among the gods themselves. He still brings us these messages in the form of dreams. As a translator of dreams, he is patron of depth psychology, therefore we can seek him when we want a deeper understanding of ourselves. In Egypt, this great power was known as Thoth, and is credited with being the source of the mystical Book of Thoth, or the tarot. He is Lord of Magic.

In the stillness of contemplation, we realize that Hermes is near us when we sense the crackle of a static charge in the air. It creates a chill up the spine. Suddenly, a slim, androgynous youth, capable of swift flight, appears. You sense something uncanny yet familiar. An orange glow pervades the atmosphere. The god, clad in winged sandals and a silvery helmet, carries a caduceus, the symbol of the human brain and nervous system. He darts and flits like quicksilver with electrically charged swiftness. His mental powers are keen and mobile. The scent of storax or perhaps lime blows in on the breeze, as monkeys and ibises congregate nearby. The temple of Hermes is a scintillating orange color, with a river of quicksilver roiling outside. As you enter you find a pair of winged sandals and a helmet for yourself. As you put them on, feel the electrical energy of Hermes course through your nerves; but the biggest charges comes when you lift his magical wand, the caduceus.

Approach Hermes with *cunning, wit,* or *humor.* Remember, the magician is also a clown!

PLANETARY OILS

Lady Sara's attributions for Mercury include the following:

AMBER RESIN OIL (*Succinum electrum*)—Healing and polarizing, it strengthens the aura and balances your masculine and feminine components; attracts sympathy and lovers and enhances telepathic powers. Blends with labdanum, castoreum, and ionones.

ANISEED OIL (*Illicium verum*)—Worn as a psychic and mental stimulant, it induces clairvoyance and energizes the brain. It has a licorice odor that mixes with sweet orange oil and coumarin. Top note.

BROOM OIL (*Spartium junceum*)—Used for healing and as a meditational aid. Its honey-rose note mixes with tuberose, cassia, mimosa, violet, and honeysuckle, as well as ionones, vetiver, and castoreum. Middle note.

CARROT SEED OIL (*Daucus carotta*)—Calming and healing, it wards off negativity. Its fatty-woody notes blend with chypres, citrus, cassia, mimosa, fougere, geranium, cedarwood, and ionones. Top note.

CHAMPACA OIL (*Michelia champaca*)—Worn as an auric energizer, it brings one's energies into harmonious balance. This warm, floral-leafy note blends into lily of the valley, carnation, rose, violet, sandalwood, and isoeugenol.

CLARY SAGE OIL (*Salvia sclarea*)—Soothing and healing, calms the nerves, excellent for meditation, may be used on the body prior to retiring for peaceful sleep. This fragrant fixative goes with labdanum, musk, coriander, cardamom, citrus, lavender, geranium, sandalwood, eugenol, and cedarwood oils. Middle note.

CYPERUS OIL (*Cyperaceae rotundus*)—Used as an aid in meditation for its calming effect. Blend with bergamot, labdanum, patchouli, and galbanum as a fixative.

FENNEL OIL (*Foeniculum dulce*)—An electric smell; used to increase one's psychic abilities. Blends into chypres and fougeres. Top note.

FENUGREEK SEED OIL (*Trigonella foenum graecum*)—Used as an anointing oil in healings. With its extreme tenacity, minute amounts can be used in oriental bases, chypres, fougeres, new-mown hay, and lavender composition.

FOUGERE OIL (*Fern*)—Used as an aid in astral projection and psychic development. It is usually bouqueted from lavender, coumarin, oakmoss, and rare woods.

HEATHER OIL (*Erica vulgaris*)—Used to heal and to promote peace, harmony, and friendliness. Use in green-herbal scents.

HONEYSUCKLE OIL (*Lonicera periclymenum*)—Used as a mental stimulant, it is also used to develop and aid intuition and psychic perception. A compounded oil of naturals and synthetics, it includes ionones, narcissus, orange, tuberose, lily, and rhodinol bases, among other ingredients.

HYACINTH OIL (*Hyacinthus orientalis*)—Used for healing, anointing, love, luck; promotes tranquility and restful sleep as well as astral projection. Compounded from cinnamic alcohol, storax, galbanum, ylang-ylang, and indoles. Top note.

LAVENDER OIL (*Lavandula vera*)—Used for healing, financial management, building energy, and promoting tranquility in relationships. Blends with bergamot, citrus, clove, oakmoss, patchouli, rosemary, clary sage, and pine. Top note.

LILAC OIL (*Syringia vulgaris*)—Aids memory and mental development, brings peace and harmony into everyday life. Compounded of ionone, indole, linalool, lillial, jasmine, rose de mai, mimosa, civet, clary sage, and ylang-ylang.

LILY OF THE VALLEY OIL (*Convallaria majalis*)—Calms the nerves and temper tantrums while promoting spiritual peace; aids restful sleep. Bouqueted from several ingredients.

LIME OIL (*Citrus medica*)—Used as a mental stimulant and energy restorer. Expressed lime oil is best for perfumery; blends with citrus, lavender, rosemary, clary sage, and amber bases. Good tenacity. Top note.

MARJORAM OIL (*Origanum majorana*)—Restores energy and is healing. For colognes, fougeres, and oriental bases. Middle note.

MASTIC OIL (*Pistacia lentiscus L.*)—Mercurial note for mental energy. Use in citrus colognes, lavender-fougeres, and straight floral bases. Top note. An electric scent.

NARCISSUS OIL (*N. jonquilla*)—Promotes peace, harmony, restful sleep, and serenity. Top note.

ORCHID OIL (*Orchidaceae*)—Aids in creativity, psychic perception, and mental clarity. Compounded with synthetics and ylang-ylang, oakmoss, vanilla, coumarin, jasmine, neroli, and tuberose.

SPIKENARD OIL (*Nardostachys jatamansi*)—Aids consciousness expansion. Blend with cedar, coumarin, ionones, labdanum, oakmoss, lavender, patchouli, pine, vetiver, ginger, and calamus.

STORAX OIL (*Liquidamber orientalis*)—Mental stimulant. Use in florals like lilac, hyacinth, carnation, violet, lavender, rose, jasmine, and ylang-ylang. Base note.

TOLU BALSAM (*Myroxylon toluiferum*)—A healing oil used in meditation. For fantasy, tabac, leather, and aldehydic perfumes; hyacinth, tuberose, gardenia, linalool, sandalwood, bergamot, labdanum, opoponax, ylang-ylang, and orange. Base note.

VALERIAN OIL (*Valeriana officinalis*)—Used in small amounts for its tranquilizing effect. Blends with patchouli, costus, oakmoss, pine, and cedar.

VIOLET OIL (*Viola odorata*)—Used to heal, ward off evil, and calm lovers' quarrels. Blends with orris, clove, ylang-ylang, sandalwood, and bergamot.

WISTERIA OIL (*Wisteria sinensis*)—An anointing oil for prayer and meditation, aids in channelling. Compounded on violet, lilac, and jasmine.

YLANG-YLANG OIL (*Canaga odorata*)—Its soothing effect is used in healing. Blends with almost all florals and synthetics; powerful, intense, tenacious. Middle note.

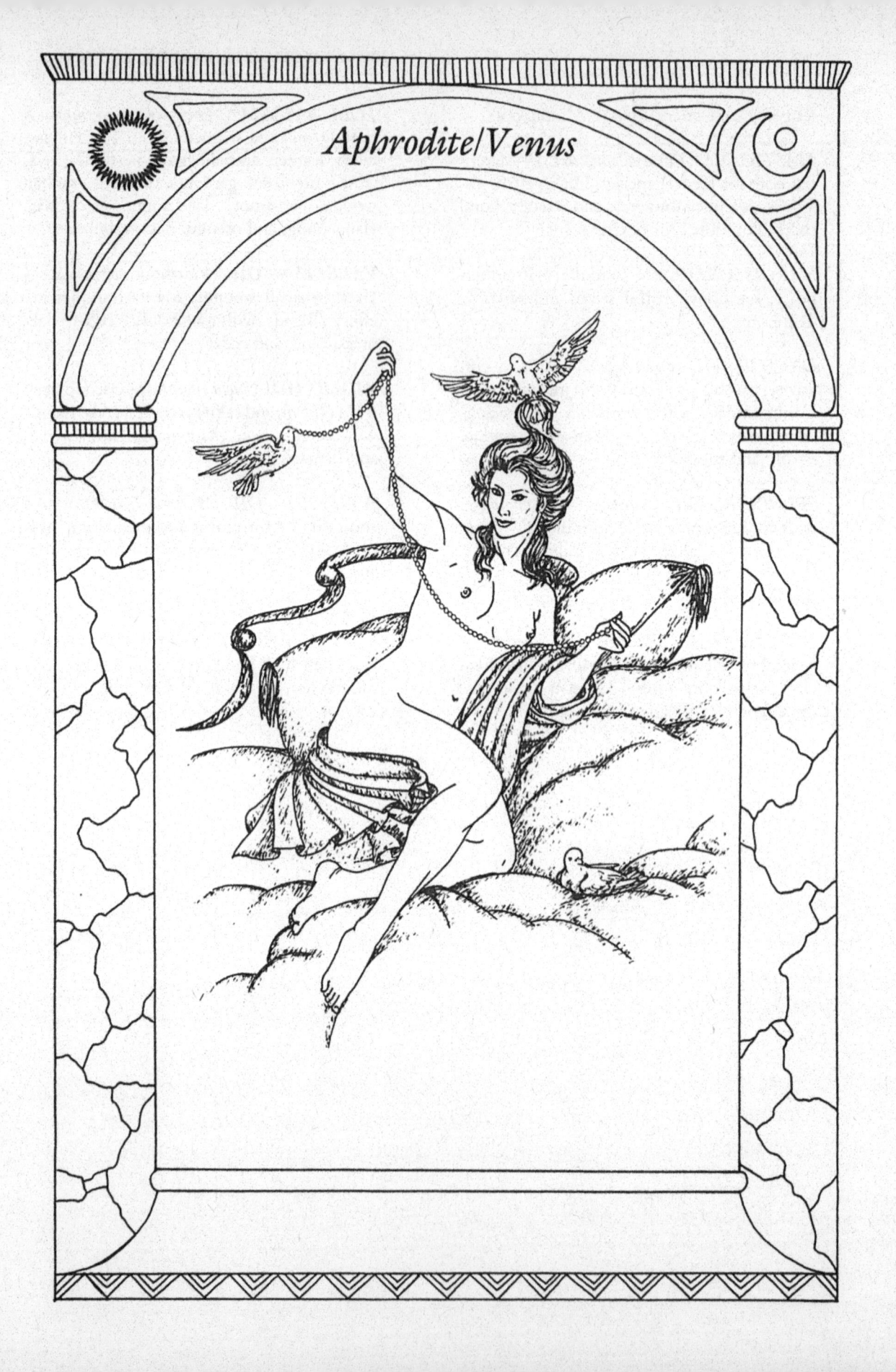

Aphrodite/Venus

VENUS = APHRODITE

It [Venus] rules sympathy, taste, likes and dislikes, attraction, magnetism, and appeal; art, beauty, aesthetic sense, comfort, pleasure, jewelry, ornaments, perfumes, luxury, and fashion.

—Larousse Encyclopedia of Astrology

ASTROLOGICAL SYMBOLISM

Venus in your chart symbolizes your need for emotional and material comfort, relationships, affinities, and values, your capacity for affection and appreciation of beauty. It represents the innate drive to unite opposites and to bring them into a state of union to achieve balance and permanent harmony. Our emotional patterns and attitudes depend largely on the position of Venus in the chart. Placement shows how we seek security, both on the emotional and material level.

Potential modes of expression for this planet include creating harmony, making peace, arriving at compromises, forming relationships, friendships, and uniting opposites. Keywords include affairs, allurement, appeal, ardor, artistry, attractiveness, collaboration, ecstasy, elegance, eroticism, enchantment, fantasy, gentleness, glamor, grace, hedonism, love, magnetism, partnership, passion, peacefulness, poise, provocativeness, rapture, seductiveness, sensuality, sexiness, sympathy, talent, and vanity.

GOD-FORM VISUALIZATION

Aphrodite, Venus, or Astarte—however she is called—is the well-known, delightful goddess of love. She is the sex symbol of the pantheon, and she lights up the morning or evening with her golden glow. Her sunny face belies the smoldering depths, her impulses can bring delight or anguish to mortals who feel her most intimate touch. The Greeks sang her praises, and her activities are recounted in several Homeric hymns:

> She went away to Cyprus, and entered her fragrant temple at Paphos, where she has a precinct and a fragrant altar. After going inside she closed the bright doors, and the Graces gave her a bath, they oiled her with sacred olive-oil, the kind that the gods always have on, that pleasant ambrosia that she was perfumed with. Having put on all her beautiful
> clothing, and having ornamented herself in gold, Aphrodite, lover of laughter, hurried away to Troy, leaving sweet-smelling Cyprus, quickly cutting a path through the clouds high up.
>
> —*The Homeric Hymns*, Charles Boer, trans.

As we close our eyes and seek Aphrodite's vision within ourselves, we first perceive the rosy dawn breaking over the sea. Out of the foaming green of the surf, a beautiful naked woman arises. With her wide hips and full body, it is immediately apparent this is no mere mortal. Her skin is supple and bronzed. She almost glows in the multicolored dawn, which is shot with rose and emerald. Walking up the beach she beckons you to join her in a nearby myrtle grove. She flashes her most alluring smile. Doves fly around her as she gathers mother-of-pearl shells along the shore. The scent of camellias, roses, and sandalwood hang langorously in the tropical air. Spring has arrived! On the far side of the myrtle bower we see a brook feeding into a pond, which contains graceful swans. In the distance we see the glint of her emerald temple with lofty spires.

Approach her with affectionate *ardor* and *sensuality*.

PLANETARY OILS

Lady Sara corresponds the following to Venus:

ALMOND OIL, BITTER (*Amygdalus amara*)—Used to create harmonious and magnetic vibrations in love and friendships. Mostly benzaldehyde, it is very volatile with no fixative. Try with anise, lilac, sweet florals. Top note.

AMYRIS OIL (*Amyris balsamifera*)—Used as a Venusian anointing oil for healing, meditation, and past-life regression. Blends with ionones, lavandin, coumarin, oakmoss, citronella, and sassafras.

ARTEMISIA OIL (*Artemisia vulgaris*)—Arouses sexual desire; restores lost virility. Gives freshness and warmth to oakmoss, patchouli, rosemary, lavender, pine, clary sage, Spanish sage, and coumarin.

BENZOIN OIL (*Styrax benzoin*)—Anointing oil; enhances beauty; purifying; worn for blessings and protection. Base note.

BIRCH OIL, SWEET (*Betula lenta*)—Generally used with other oils for love or sexual attraction blends. A wintergreen note.

BOIS DE SIAM OIL (*Cunninghamina sinensis*)—Used as a meditation and anointing oil.

CAMELLIA OIL (*Camellia sasanqua*)—Makes the wearer unforgettable. A compounded oil using linalool, ylang-ylang, isoeugenol, jasmine, orange, and musk.

CARDAMOM OIL (*Elettoria cardamomum*)—A magnetic essence for sexual attraction known as Fire of Venus. Blend into muguet and rose bases; use with bergamot, olibanum, ylang-ylang, labdanum, cedar, neroli, coriander. Middle note.

CITRONELLA OIL (*Cymbopogon nardus*)—Attracts new customers or friends; maintains serenity in the home; wards off evil and negativity. Mostly an industrial perfume. Top note.

CORIANDER OIL (*Coriandrum sativum*)—Aphrodisiac; oil of attraction. Blend with anise, cardamom, bergamot, jasmine, lilac, olibanum, cinnamon, citrus, sandalwood, and cypress oil. Top note.

CUMIN OIL (*Cuminum cyminum*)—For peace and harmony and insuring fidelity in one's mate. Blend with lavender, rosemary, galbanum, oakmoss, bois de rose. Top note.

GALBANUM OIL (*Ferula galbaniflua*)—A spiritual, purifying oil for ritual. Blend with coumarin, oakmoss, pine, storax, violet, narcissus, and gardenia. Base note.

LABDANUM OIL (*Cistus creticus L.*)—A slightly narcoticlike, magnetic fragrance. Blends with citrus, clary sage, oakmoss, juniper, lavender, pine, opoponax, and synthetic musks. Base note.

LOVAGE OIL (*Livisticum officinale*)—Increases magnetism or sensual appeal, but has very limited use in perfumery because of its celerylike smell.

ORRIS OIL (*Iris florentina*)—Worn to attract the opposite sex. Good in delicate florals like violet, mimosa, cyclamen, freesia, and orchid. Middle note.

PEPPERMINT OIL (*Mentha piperita*)—Clears the mind, calms the nerves; dispels the bad and attracts good things. Use in lavender colognes and fougere. Top note.

ROSE OIL (*Rose centifolia, Rosa damascena*)—Induces thoughts of loving affection; peaceful harmonious vibrations; an anointing oil for symbolic objects. Blends well with florals, especially jasmine. Top note.

SANDALWOOD OIL (*Santalum album*)—Spiritual essence for healing, prayer, meditation, and past-life regression. Goes with amber, opoponax, precious woods, oakmoss, labdanum, patchouli, artificial musks, vetiver, and ionones. Base note.

TONKA BEAN OIL (*Dipteryx odorata*)—Used for healing and attracting good fortune. Tonka absolute is preferred with lavender, clary sage, storax, heliotropine, bergamot, oakmoss, and other esters. Base note.

VANILLA OIL (*Vanilla planifolia*)—Used for soothing, healing, good luck, and "love" blends. Tincture is best for perfumery. Base note.

VERBENA OIL (*Verbena triphylla*)—A stimulant for mental creativity that also dispels negativity or evil. Blend with citrus, neroli, heliotropine, ionones, nitromusks, spice oils, elemi, olibanum, and tolu. Middle note.

Ares/Mars

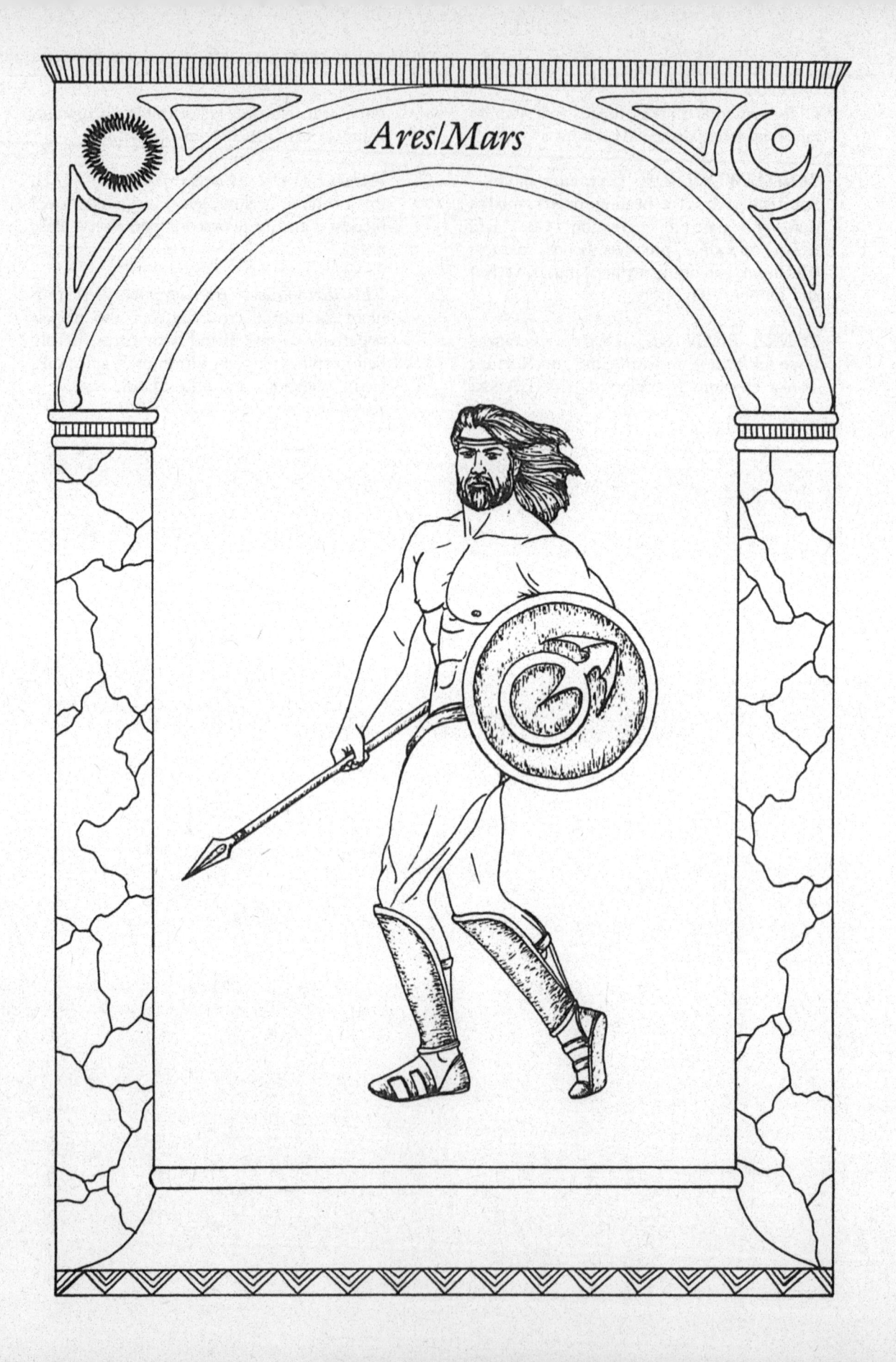

It [Mars] rules the sex drive, the muscles, the appetite, the sense of smell, the voice, the breath, the prana or vital energy, as well as steel, knives, weapons, and fire.

—*Larousse Encyclopedia of Astrology*

MARS = ARES

ASTROLOGICAL SYMBOLISM

Mars is the extroverted form of the instinct for self-defense or self-preservation. It also symbolizes your desire to prove yourself, and the mode you choose will depend on what sign and house Mars occupies in your natal chart. The position of Mars at your birth determines how you use your energy and where you make your presence felt.

Keywords include ambition, ardent desire, assertion, bravery, courage, discipline, executive ability, fitness, goal-directed energy, obedience, robustness, sex drive, strength, valor, and zeal.

GOD-FORM VISUALIZATION

We generally consider Ares or Mars to be a quarrelsome troublemaker, but let's not forget we can invoke the higher qualities of this planet for courage and peace (both peace of mind and war-preventing world peace). Mankind has called on him from earliest times, as this Homeric hymn to Ares shows:

Hear me,
helper of mankind,
dispenser of youth's sweet courage,
beam down from up there
your gentle light
on our lives,
and your martial power,
so that I can shake off
cruel cowardice
from my head,
and diminish that deceptive rush
of my spirit, and restrain
that shrill voice in my heart
that provokes me
to enter the chilling din of battle.
You happy god,
give me courage,
let me linger
in the safe laws of peace,
and thus escape
from battles with enemies
and the fate of a violent death.
—*The Homeric Hymns*, Charles Boer, trans.

Looking through the dust kicked up by the fracas, we see Ares approaching us through the din of battle, emerging from strife and war, furious with the adrenaline of battle pumping through him. Combat has reinforced his unmanageable personality; he is obstinate. Pausing to rest, he binds his wounds with arnica for protection and barberry for strength. Like a wolf or a bear, he does not shrink from conflict. His color is blood-red, and has been repeatedly soaked in the ruby liquid. He climbs atop his chariot to stable his weary horses. The burliest, bearded warrior in heavy bronze armor with a tall-crested helmet, he threatens us good-naturedly with his enormous spear. After checking the status of the battle he retires to his tent for renewal. Scorned as a barbaric warlord for his bravura and violent, aggressive nature, Ares seeks solace in the accepting arms of the beautiful Aphrodite. She finds his powerful arms, mighty heart, virility, and roughly passionate embrace irresistible. After all, there is *something* about a military man!

Approach him through *courage*; don't let aggression or anger possess you.

PLANETARY SCENTS

Lady Sara's choices for Mars include:

ALLSPICE OIL (*Pimenta officinalis*)—A warm scent, worn to strengthen the will, energize, and vitalize.

AMMONIACUM OIL (*Dorena ammoniacum*)—Worn for protection and purification and as an anointing oil for exorcism. A balsamic fixative.

ARNICA FLOWER OIL (*Arnica montana*)—A protective anointing oil for channels. Use in colognes, herbaceous types, chypres, fougere, tabac, leather. Base note.

ASAFETIDA OIL (*Ferula foetida*)—Used for purification and protection. Its garlic-onion top note gives way to a rich, sweet balsamic body note.

BARBERRY OIL (*Berberis vulgaris*)—Strengthens both will and body. The odor recalls a lily-rose combination with an anise and indole undertone.

BASIL OIL (*Ocimum basilicum*)—Used for purification, protection, and exorcism. Blend with opoponax, bergamot, clary sage, oakmoss, and lime.

CACTUS FLOWER OIL (*Cactus grandiflorus*)—Worn for increasing mental clarity and psychic perception. Smells like a vanilla-rose-jasmine blend.

CALAMUS OIL (*Acorus calamus*)—Its mind-altering effect is used for meditation and psychic development. Use in woody-orientals, leathers, and amber bases with cinnamon, labdanum, olibanum, patchouli, ionones, nitro musks, and cedarwood. Middle note.

CANELLA OIL (*Canella alba*)—Anointing oil for healing, strengthening, and vitalizing the aura. Usually compounded of cinnamon, and clove.

GERANIUM OIL (*Pelargonium fragrans*)—For ritual baths and purification and good fortune or assistance. Used extensively in perfumery as rhodinol. Middle note.

GINGER OIL (*Zingiber officinale*)—A hot scent, used as a psychic, physical, and sexual energizer. Blend with bois de rose, cedar, coriander, coumarin, citrus, eugenol, and musk.

OPOPANAX OIL (*Commiphora erythroea*)—Worn for protection and purification. Blends with clary sage, coriander, labdanum, heavy floral, and leather. Base note.

PATCHOULI OIL (*Pogostemon patchouli*)—Wards off evil and negativity; facilitates peaceful separations. Blends with labdanum, vetiver, sandalwood, ionones, cedar, coumarin, oakmoss, geranium, clove, rose, citrus, and musks. Base note.

PINE, SCOTCH OIL (*Pinus sylvestris*)—Aids healing by cleansing the aura and soothing the nerves. Blend with rosemary, cedar, citrus, coumarin, oakmoss.

SNAKEROOT, CANADIAN OIL (*Asarum canadense*)—Purifying, protecting oil for anointing oneself to stimulate the psychic centers. Use with bergamot, costus, ionones, oakmoss, patchouli, pine, clary sage, and selected florals.

TOBACCO FLOWER OIL (*Nicotiana affinis*)—Promotes physical vitality. Compounded with clary sage, tonka, rose, carnation, honey, labdanum, and olibanum.

TOBACCO LEAF OIL (*Nicotiana affinis*)—Worn for physical vitality. Blend with sandalwood, castoreum, labdanum, clary sage, vetiver, bergamot, and cedar.

WORMWOOD OIL (*Artemisia absinthium*)—Worn by trance mediums to aid in evocations. Blend with oakmoss, jasmine, orange-flower, and hyacinth. Top note.

Zeus/Jupiter

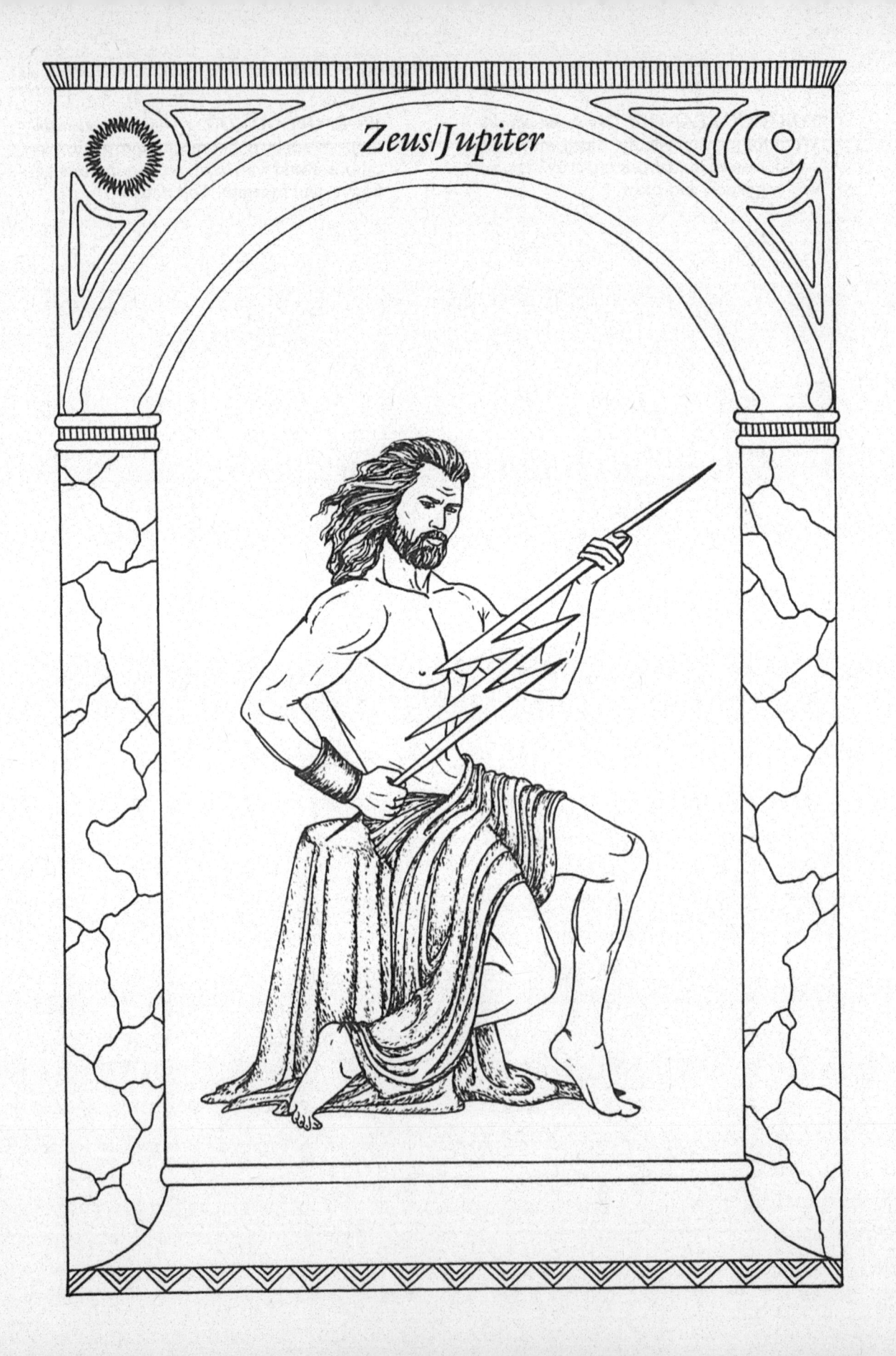

> *Zeus is the head of the Olympian gods and belongs to the trinity of the father/authority principle with his brothers Poseidon and Hades. As the ultimate authority he comes closest to embodying the archetype of the Self.*
>
> —Philo Stone, *Pantheon*

JUPITER = ZEUS

ASTROLOGICAL SYMBOLISM

Jupiter exemplifies our philosophical, spiritual, and religious needs as well as our desires to extend ourselves to others, expand our horizons, and propagate ourselves. The position of Jupiter in the natal chart tells us how we experience our need for connection to divinity, or the Creator. It reveals our optimal direction for growth and expansion of personal horizons. It can also characterize our metaphysical perspective, or world-view.

Positive modes of expression include illumination, growth of consciousness and insight, increase of knowledge as well as understanding, mercy, the formation of spiritual and religious values, furthering one's own projects and insights, and improving one's social status. Keywords are achievement, authority, decisiveness, dynamism, energy, enthusiasm, equitability, extraversion, faith, good fortune, generosity, geniality, idealism, independence, joviality, leniency, luck, magnificence, optimism, nobility, political savvy, prosperous, respectability, self-assurance, success, wise judgment, and wholeness.

GOD-FORM VISUALIZATION

Zeus, as the king of the gods, incorporates all of their qualities within his own expansive wholeness. He is an integrated personality with high well-being, nobility, and tremendous success. We can think of him as the chairman of the board at Mount Olympus.

Relaxing, we contemplate the figure of Zeus with the eye of the mind, initially seeing brilliant flashes of lightning in the inner sky. As the clouds part and our eyes adjust to the radiant light, we see the regal Zeus in his splendid palace. The sovereign's throne is solid lapis lazuli, shot through with gold. He is surrounded by the other deities who have assembled at his court. The palace is exquisite, with its giant columns forming an open structure that allows for free circulation. Eagles fly freely about, coming and going as they wish. The various appointments of the palace-temple are in royal blue, deep purple, and gold. Cedarwood figures prominently in the construction of the audience room and also burns as fragrant incense. Approaching the dais cautiously, we see that the monarch himself is awesome. A large, muscular, aristocratic figure, he lounges calmly, surveying his domain while drinking ambrosia from a huge amethyst goblet. Suddenly, we feel lit up, from both without and within. Are these bursts of lightning and thunder actually penetrating to the core of our being to bring mystical illumination? As we feel penetrated by his majesty, power, and glory, we realize that Zeus is the divine generative or impregnating force on the spiritual level.

Approach him with *reverence* and *awe*, and never demand that he reveal his full glory to you, lest you be blasted by its magnitude.

PLANETARY OILS

Lady Sara's selected fragrances for Jupiter include:

ALOE WOOD OIL (Aquilaria Agallocha)—Worn for protection and healing. Known as agar oil, it blends with vetiver, sandalwood, geranium, and linalool.

ARAUCARIA OIL (Callitropsis araucarioides)—Attracts success; dispels evil; facilitates attraction, love, harmony, and friendship. Blend with clary sage, methylionones, linalool, fougere, lily, and lilac. Middle note.

BALM MELISSA OIL (Melissa officinalis)—Helps fulfill wishes for success, friendship, and money. Use with citrus and herbaceous blends. Middle note.

BUCHU OIL (Barosma venusta)—Worn for blessings, protection, and astral healing. Used for chypre and certain types of colognes.

CANADA BALSAM (Abies balsamea)—Enhances powers during ritual; wards off evil. A fixative for pine fragrances.

CARNATION OIL (Dianthus caryophylis)—Used for anointing, healing, and energizing. Blend with rose, lily, narcissus, lavender, ylang-ylang, clary sage, and castoreum.

CASCARILLA OIL (Croton eleuteria)—Boosts energy and power for rituals and healing. Blend with nutmeg, pepper, dalmatian sage, oakmoss, and cedar. Middle note.

CEDARWOOD OIL (Juniperus virginiana)—Enhances honor, wealth, and dignity. Blend with vetiver, sandalwood, and patchouli. Top note.

CLOVER BLOSSOM OIL (Trefle)—Used to attract success and luck. A compounded oil.

COUMARIN OIL (Liatris idoratissima)—Promotes attraction, friendship, and love. Tonka absolute contains up to 45% coumarin; it goes with lavender, clary sage, cinnamates, storax, bergamot, oakmoss, and heliotropine. Base note.

DAVANA OIL (Artemisia pallens)—For ritual anointing, blessing, and healing. Blends with chypre and fougere materials such as oakmoss and labdanum.

EVERLASTING OIL (Helichrysum augustifolium)—For anointing, blessing, and meditation. Mix with coumarin, lavender, clary sage, citrus, linalool, rose, Peru balsam, and clove.

FIR BALSAM OIL (Abies balsamea)—An aid in meditation, it is also used for rituals concerning nature spirits. Blends with coumarin, oakmoss, citrus, rosemary, juniper berry, labdanum, patchouli, and lavandin.

HYSSOP OIL (Hyssopus officinalis)—Assures faithfulness of friends and lovers, financial success, purification, and protection during exorcism. Goes with citrus, lavender, rosemary, myrtle, laurel, clary sage, and linalool. Middle note. (Horsey smell)

MIGNONETTE OIL (Reseda odorata)—Soothing and harmonizing, it restores body and soul. Reseda is from Egypt and smells like violet leaves.

MONARDA OIL (Monarda didyma)—A psychic energizer. Monarda didyma smells somewhat like lavender and ambergris.

NUTMEG OIL (Myristica fragrans)—Brings luck in all areas and protects from all evil. Blend with oakmoss, bay, linalool, lavender, and coumarin.

OAKMOSS OIL (Evernia prunastri)—Energizer, especially for working with nature spirits. Fixative for many combinations. Base note.

PERU BALSAM OIL (*Myroxylon pereirae*)—Attracts success and prosperity. Fixative for floral, balsamic, and spicy notes; blends with araucaria, and sandalwood, gardenia, tuberose, carnation, rose, and ylang-ylang.

SAGE OIL (*Salvia officinalis*)—Used for cleansing, healing, and restoring energy. Powerful top note, with tenacious sweet-herbaceous smell for mixing with lavender, rosemary, citrus, and bois de rose.

Hera/Saturn

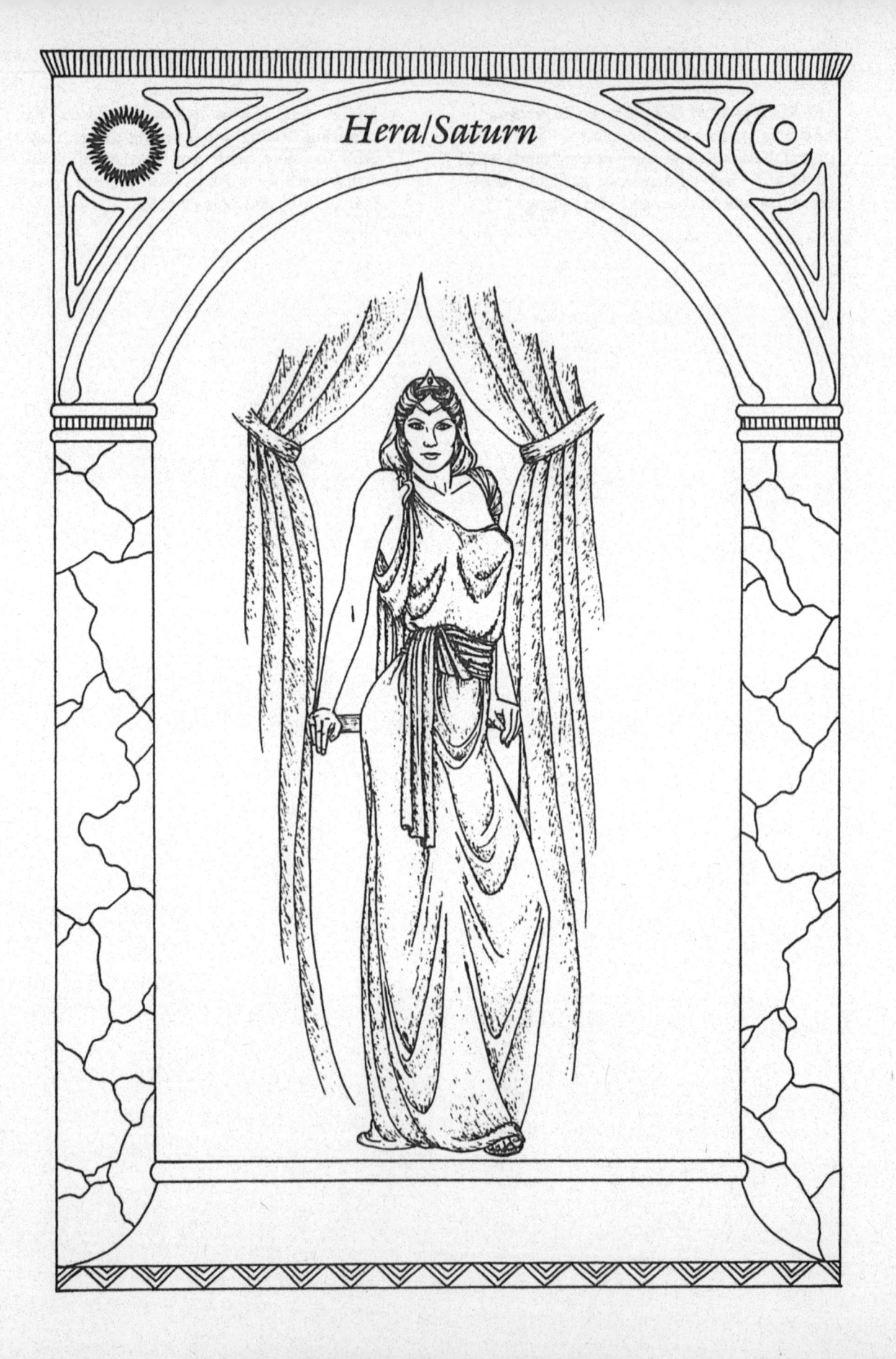

In mythology the lily was consecrated to Juno because it was alleged that "from the milk of her breasts sprang this beautiful flower."

SATURN = HERA

ASTROLOGICAL SYMBOLISM

Saturn represents not only our ability to bring great energy to bear on a situation but also our limitations in that regard—it is our limiting self-definition that restricts consciousness. Saturn shows how we can learn even through painful experience. According to astrologer Robert Hand, Saturn has the greatest effect on a person in a social context, it directs our attention outside of ourselves. It is the pragmatic reality of structure and form. Saturn shows us where we need disciplined work, symbolizing an innate desire for ego development and personal and social responsibility. We find our limits by testing them, experiencing vulnerability, and re-shaping our character despite suffering and disappointment.

Keywords include ambition, aristocracy, capability, competence, conservatism, control, diligence, discipline, fidelity, goal-orientation, guidance, introspection, order, patience, perseverance, pillar of society, practicality, pragmatism, regulation, responsibility, self-esteem, sobriety, structure, super-ego, and tenacity.

GOD-FORM VISUALIZATION

God-forms that correspond to this planet are of two types. The first is the "grandfather time" god—Saturn, Chronos, Yahweh, or Brahma. The second partakes of the feminine principle and is exemplified by Hera, or Juno, the celestial queen. She represents, among other things, the mating instinct, marriage and divorce, and the sacred marriage, or *hierosgamos*. Hera embodies our yearning to be a spouse, feeling essentially incomplete without a partner. This goddess seeks to realize herself through our marriages. In her own way, she is the equal of her spouse, Zeus.

Breathing deeply of her perfumes, we begin to invoke Hera. We see a royal blue mist, which parts to reveal a sumptuous temple-palace. These spacious quarters open onto a courtyard with pomegranate trees. Peacocks and cuckoo birds roam freely about. Suddenly, the stately queen of the sky steps forth with her retinue of courtiers. She seats herself at her dressing table and begins to groom herself meticulously for her public duties. Her heirloom jewelry includes a large star sapphire ring surrounded by pearls. It was probably a gift from her creative son, the smith Hephaistos.

She perfumes herself with civet oil to please her husband; sometimes she employs magnolia, myrrh, or other oils to bring peace and harmony and dispel discord in her matrimonial life. She seems a young but rather mature woman of severe beauty. As "woman deified" she always wears her diadem or a high crown of cylindrical shape when in public. When she sheds her long tunic for her husband, she envelops herself modestly in her long veil, revealing only her nobility and desire to please her husband. Approach this noble one with great *deference*.

PLANETARY OILS

Some of Lady Sara's selections for Saturn follow.

BERGAMOT OIL (*Citrus bergamia*)—Anointing oil for protection from misfortune and physical danger. Blends in florals such as muguet, chypre, gardenia, lavender, and violet. Top note.

BORONIA OIL (*Boronia megastigma*)—Expands consciousness and crystallizes creative thoughts. Blend with clary sage, bergamot, costus, sandalwood, and linalool.

CASTOREUM OIL (*Castor fiber*)—A base for Saturnian fragrances. Blends with amber, calamus, cananga, cedar, chamomile, labdanum, oakmoss, and sandalwood. Base note.

CIVET OIL (*Viverra civetta*)—Brings protection, enlightenment, and sexual magnetism. Mix with nitro musks, coumarin, and vanilla. Fixative.

COSTUS OIL (*Aplotaxis lappa*)—Makes one attractive, sensual, and magnetic. Expensive; use small amounts with cinnamic alcohol, nitro musks, patchouli, opoponax, and oakmoss.

CYPRESS OIL (*Cypress sempervirens*)—Brings healing, luck, and financial gain. Anoint yourself for blessing and protection. Blend with juniper berry, pine, and citrus. Base note.

DATURA FLOWER OIL (*Datura stramonium*)—One of the most sensually magnetic of all oils.

LILY OF THE VALLEY OIL (*Convallaria majalis*)—Used for restful sleep and to ease heartache. Muguet is compounded from jasmine, linalool, and terpineol.

MAGNOLIA OIL (*Magnolia grandiflora*)—Lends peace and harmony to meditation and spiritual development. Compounded of jasmine, neroli, rose, and ionone.

MYRRH OIL (*Commiphora myrrha*)—Sacred anointing oil for blessing, protection, meditation, and healing. See "Binah." Top note.

> *Cronus reached out with his left hand and seized his father, and with his right he castrated him. . . . Blood gushed forth upon Earth, and from it in due course she bore the Furies and the Giants, and the Ash nymphs, from whom the gods made the third race of men, the Bronze men . . . an ash plantation can by suitable management . . . be made to yield a supply of tough, strait, strong stems for spear shafts . . . and the regular pruning may have contributed something to the myth of castration.*
>
> —John Pinsent, *Greek Mythology*

URANUS = URANUS

ASTROLOGICAL SYMBOLISM

The energy of Uranus is iconoclastic—it breaks up the old and makes way for radical re-vision. It is associated with alternative states of consciousness and enlightenment, the harbinger of change and new experiences. It fosters detachment and the desire to break free. Contact with this mind-oriented planetary energy helps us to reestablish contact with the living self.

Keywords include genius, imagination, independence, originality, insight, intuition, inventiveness, originality, and unconventionality.

GOD-FORM VISUALIZATION

Uranus is best visualized as the starry heavens with its multitudes of galaxies, nebulas, and vast expanses.

PLANETARY OILS

Lady Sara recommends the following for Uranus:

AMBER RESIN OIL (*Succinum electrum*)—Healing and polarizing, it also strengthens the aura and brings inner polarities into harmonious balance. Blend with castoreum, labdanum, and ionones; use in leather bases and colognes.

AMBRETTE OIL (*Hibiscus abelmoschus*)—Worn for sensual magnetism and stimulation. Mix with rose, neroli, sandalwood, and cyclamen. Middle note.

ATRACTYLIS OIL (*Atractylis lancea*)—Promotes astral projection and prophetic dreaming. Fixative with vetiver, ionones, isoeugenol, opoponax, and nitro musks. Leather note: atractylis, isoeugenol, phenylethylalcohol.

BROOM OIL (*Cytisus scoparius*)—For healing and astral projection. Melds with ionones, vetiver, castoreum, green notes, tabac, and aldehydes. Middle note.

CURCUMA OIL (*Curcuma Longa*)—Used to anoint the soles of the feet for protection during rituals. Blend with cistus oil, cananga, elecampane, ginger, labdanum, orris, ionones, nitro musks, and heliotropine.

ELEMI OIL (*Canarium luzonicum*)—Used to anoint the chakras, it enhances psychism. Fixative for citrus, bergamot, verbena, and lavender colognes. Top note.

MUSK OIL (*Moschus moschiferus*)—Stimulates self-confidence, reliance, determination; enhances extroversion and the will. Sexual stimulant. Goes with a variety of bases, including oriental, heavy-floral, aldehydic, muguet, rose, clover, and violet. Base note.

NEROLI OIL (*Neroli bigarade*)—Rubbed on arms and legs for sexual magnetism, to attract love and romance. Classic in cologne, blends with citrus, synthetics, and most florals with its orange smell.

Uranus

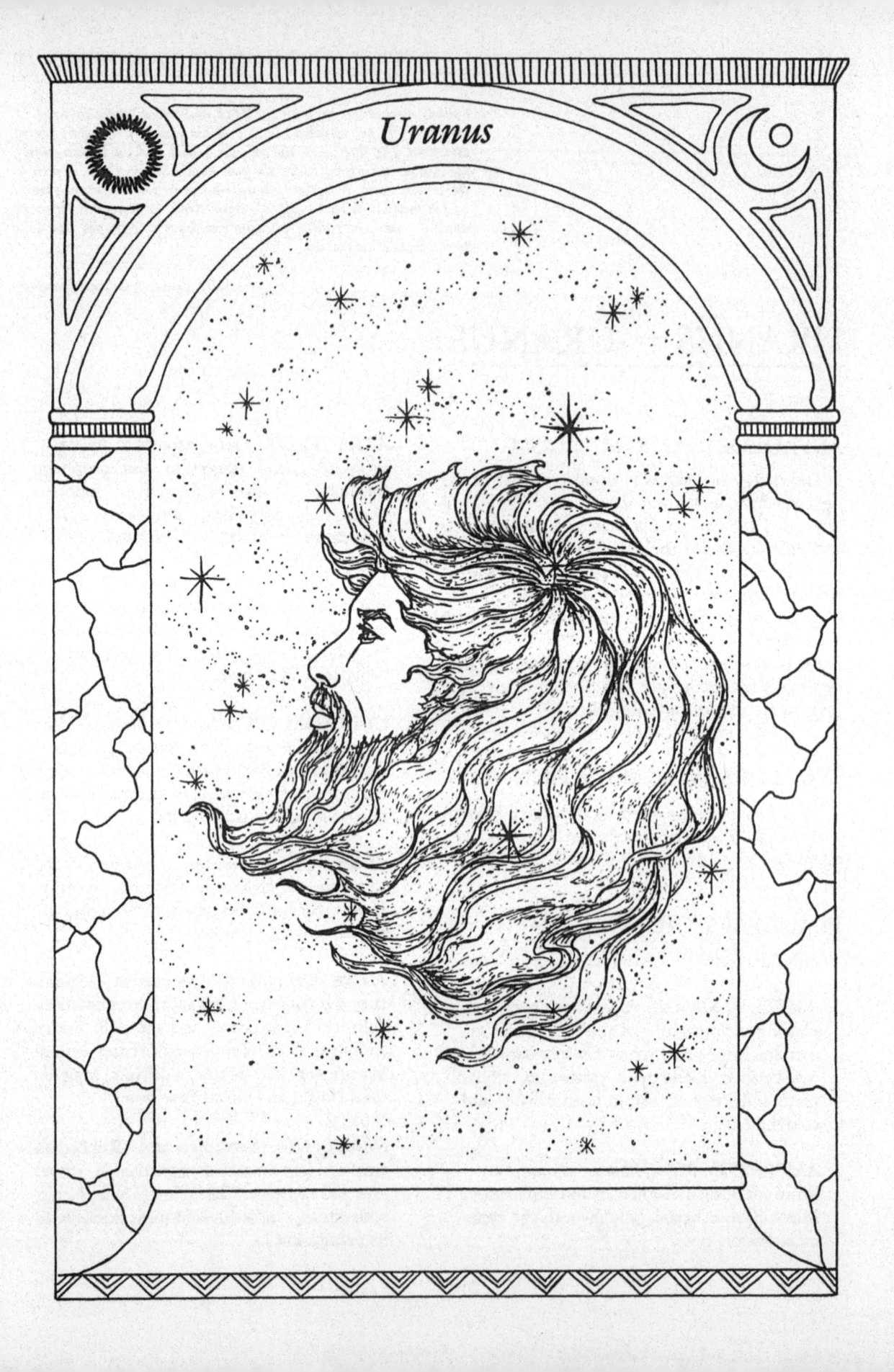

RUE OIL (*Ruta graveolens*)—For uncrossing and psychic self-defense. Can irritate the skin and mucous membranes, so don't wear it. Top note.

SIBERIAN FIR OIL (*Abies sibirica*)—Promotes serenity and meditation; used as anointing oil for healings; helps contact nature spirits. Blends with pine and other fir-needle oils, coumarin, oakmoss, nitro musks, citrus, juniper, labdanum patchouli, and lavender.

SUMBUL OIL (*Ferula sumbul*)—Sensually magnetic, it binds another's love. Fixative for orientals, musk, and precious wood bases. Rare oil.

SYRINGA OIL (*Philadelphia coronarius*)—Attracts romance. Floral and amber.

Poseidon/Neptune

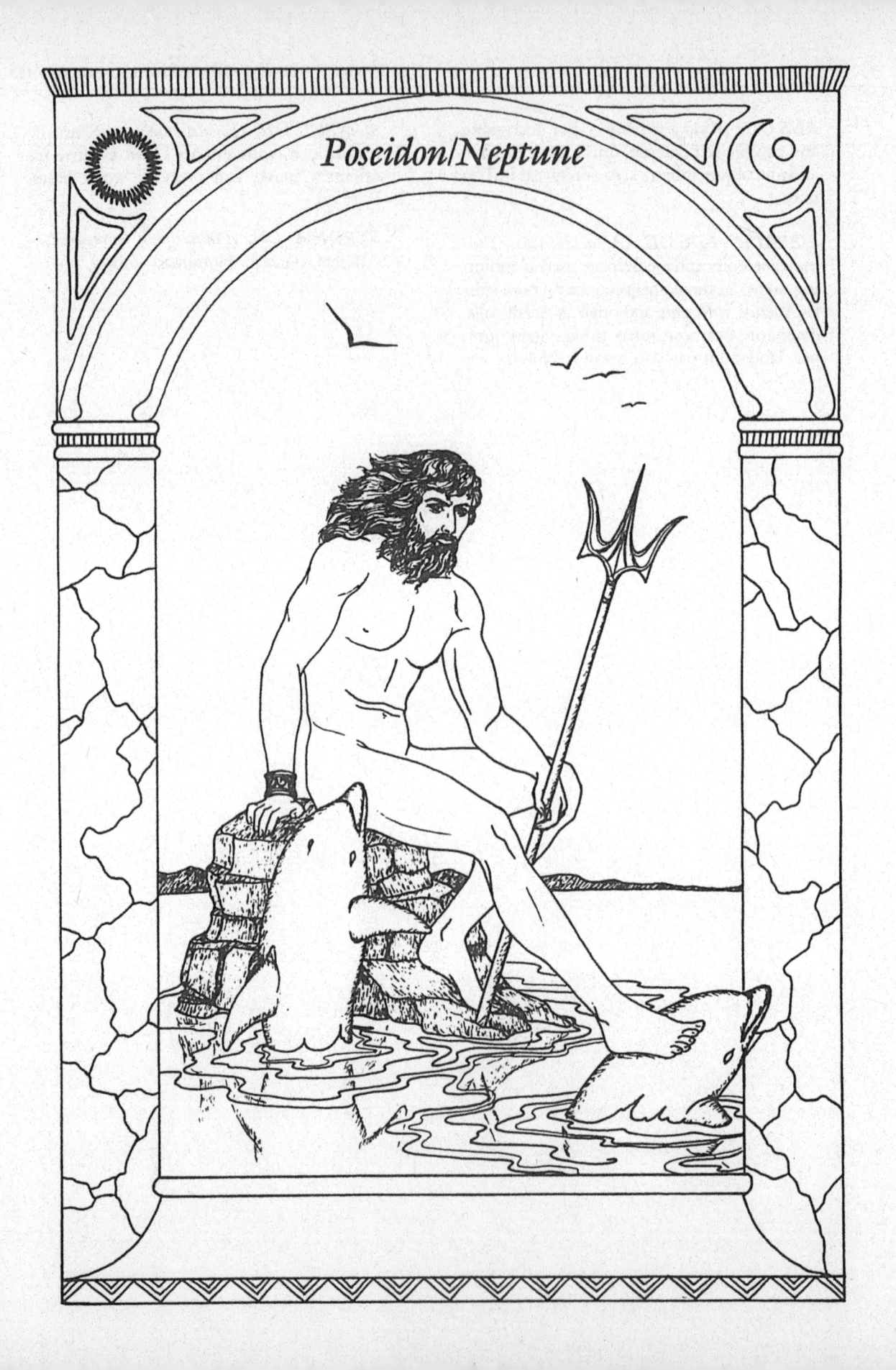

> *For the alchemists, Neptune was quite simply a symbol for water.... The discovery of psychoanalysts that the ocean is a symbol of the unconscious, has, at the same time, proved beyond question the relationship of Neptune with the deepest layers of the individual, and the universal, soul.... He is king of the deeps of the subconscious and of the turbulent waters of life.*
>
> —J.E. Cirlot, *A Dictionary of Symbols*

NEPTUNE = POSEIDON

ASTROLOGICAL SYMBOLISM

The planetary powers conferred by Neptune include psychism and artistic creativity. Contact with Neptunian energy opens the door to a universe of unlimited possibilities—even the attainment of nirvana, merging the personality in infinite being and consciousness. But beware, since Neptune can also bring illusions, confusion, and crisis, as well as ideals, truth, and divinity of mystical experience.

Keywords include compassion, elusiveness, fantasy, idealism, impressionability, mystery, self-sacrifice, spirituality, subtlety, and universality.

GOD-FORM VISUALIZATION

Poseidon is not only the king of the sea, he also rules over earthquakes, which are one of his modes of manifestation.

Taking three deep breaths, and seeking the image of Poseidon within, we see the aquamarine ocean covered with pearlescent foam. Suddenly the sea parts widely, waves billowing in opposite directions. From the depths, like a vast upwelling sigh, Poseidon vaults forth from his splendid undersea palace. He glides across the waves in his mighty chariot, barely touching the water, like a hydroplane. He is escorted everywhere by dolphins and darting schools of fish. The scent of ambergris from sperm whales mingles with the salty sting of the surf. From his beryl- and barnacle-encrusted craft, he exudes the power of a masterful presence. He is not serene but dynamically majestic. He thrusts out his bare chest more often than his trident in a display of his masculinity. His thick beard and disorderly black hair look as though he had just emerged from a swim. On shore, Poseidon is still a mighty power—the horsemaster par excellence. His horses are the finest anywhere and gladly display their obedience. As he rides off into the distance, his steeds shake the earth with their thundering hooves.

Approach him with a sense of profound *self-surrender* to upwelling instincts.

PLANETARY OILS

Lady Sara's offering for Neptune include:

AMBERGRIS OIL (sperm whale)—A sexual attractant and energizer. A fixative that has no particular scent of its own yet enhances others. Base note.

CYPERUS OIL (*Cyperaceae rotundus*)—Balances and harmonizes holistically to increase spiritual awareness. Blends with mimosa, cassie, costus, methylionones, isoeugenol, oakmoss, and clary sage.

FOUGERE OIL (Fern)—Enhances spiritual awakening and psychic development. Compounded largely of oakmoss, coumarin, and amyl salicylate.

HELICHRYSUM OIL (*Helichrysum angustifolium*)—Also called *everlasting* or *immortelle*, this spiritual oil expands your perceptions on the inner planes. Blend it with boronia, chamomile, citrus, geraniol, ionones, labdanum, neroli, lavender, mimosa, oakmoss, orris, and clary sage.

SYRINGA OIL (*Philadelphus coronarius*)—Allegedly opens the third eye, enhancing spiritual development. Blend into jasmine, amber, and cassia bases.

Hades/Pluto

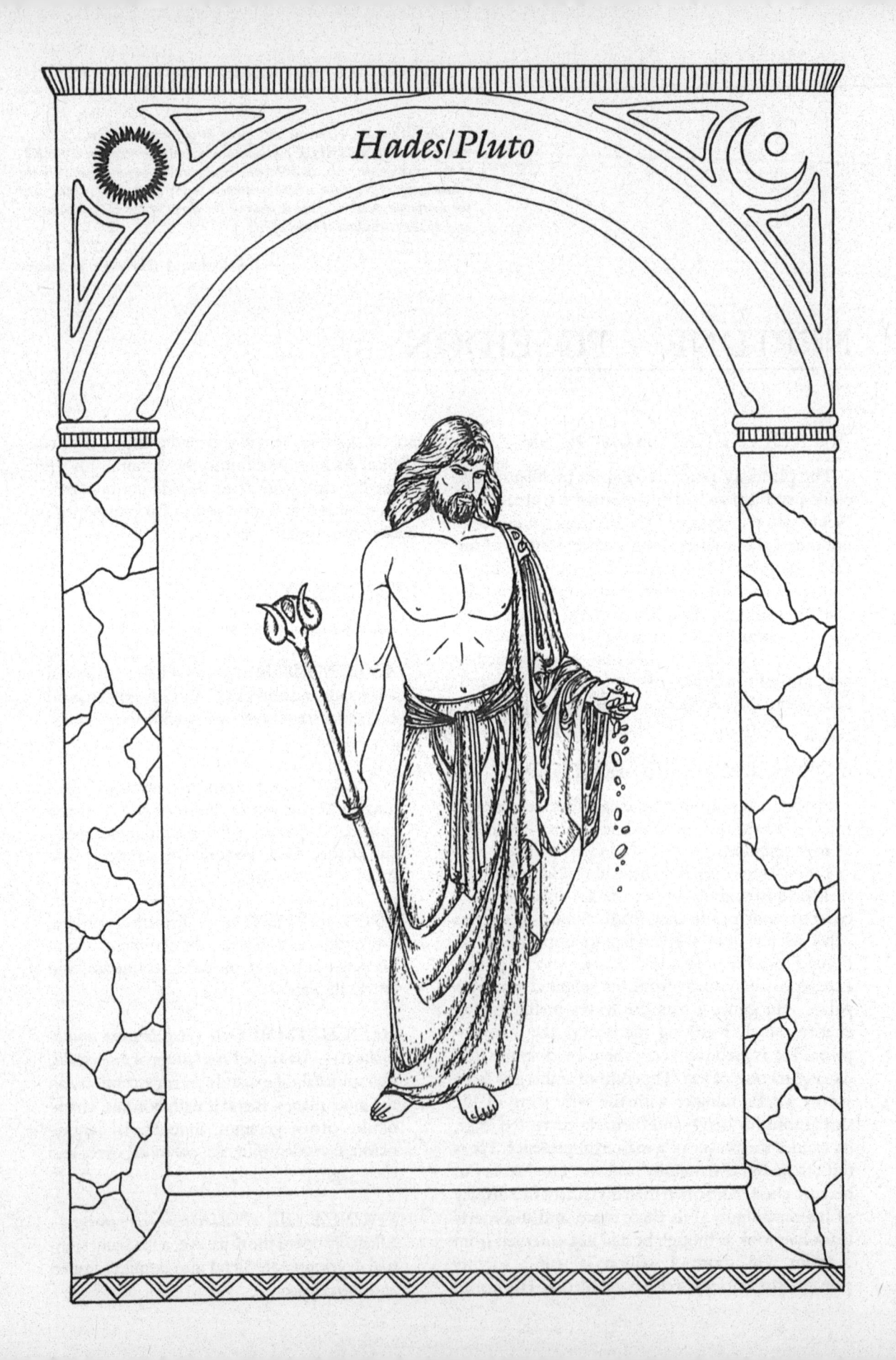

> *Gaia had approved the marriage and sent up flowers that tempted Persephone down a secluded valley which either led to Hades or where Hades raped her (flowers are the proper accompaniment of a sacred marriage, and Gaia has specially created the narcissus which like Koré returns in the spring) and from which he carried her off.*
>
> —John Pinsent, *Greek Mythology*

PLUTO = HADES

ASTROLOGICAL SYMBOLISM

As the archetype of death and rebirth, Pluto symbolizes the most radical transformations of consciousness. Through breakdowns in ordinary reality, Pluto teaches the necessity for detachment. Pluto also symbolizes the transcendental aspect of sexuality, the evolutionary power of the life and death cycle of the body. But the soul can also experience death, decay, and subsequent resurrection.

Keywords include charisma, power, regeneration, renewal, sexual magnetism, surrender to change, and wealth.

GOD-FORM VISUALIZATION

Pluto, the Greek Hades, is the king of the underworld, the realm not only of death but of the deepest subconscious. He is known as the Wealthy One, both because of his treasure of departed souls and because of the symbolic treasures entombed in the deepest recesses of human awareness.

Closing our eyes we depart from the realm of ordinary awareness on a short journey that takes us far from the land of the living. At the most remote reaches of our awareness we enter a cave so deep it seems to penetrate to the very center of the earth. There we find vast caverns, whipped by winds of unknown source. In this cold, gray land we can sometimes think we perceive phantoms drifting and floating in the swirling vapors. The sighing of the winds mingle with the ghostly wailing. Shortly after, we come upon a vast chamber from which comes a glow that flashes like opal. It has a pungent smell that does little to allay our sense of terror and mystery. Not daring to meet death face to face, we peek in to see the reflective shadow of an enormous form. We know from this shadow that he has the head of an immense black ram, who is the king of the underworld in human form. This encounter with death strikes deeply into our hearts, and we are transformed at the root of our being, so far from consciousness that we remain unaware of the change. Having been granted this boon, we depart for sunnier realms.

Approach Hades obliquely, with *fear* and *trembling*; do not face him directly.

PLANETARY OILS

Lady Sara attributes aspects of the following scents to Pluto:

BOUVARDIA OIL
BEGONIA OIL
DATURA FLOWER OIL
OPOPONAX OIL
STEPHANOTIS OIL
AMBROSIA OIL
LABDANUM OIL
AMBERGRIS OIL

She does not elaborate on them further, since there are "no ancient or traditional correspondences or attributions." She feels it best for students to experiment and find those essences that share a hidden harmony with Pluto in their mind's eye.

SUPPLIERS

UNITED STATES

American Aromatics, Inc.
    1295 Northern Blvd.
    Manhasset, NY 11030
Aphrodisia Products, Inc.
    45 Washington St.
    Brooklyn, NY 11201
Aroma Resources,
    Div. Biddle Sawyer Corp.
    2 Penn Plaza, Suite 2355
    New York, NY 10121
Atlanta Fragrance, Inc.
    984 Industrial Park Dr.
    Marietta, GA 30062
Attar Herbs & Spices, Inc.
    Playground Road
    New Ipswich, NH 03071
Auro Trading
    18 A Hangar Way
    Watsonville, CA 95076
Auroma Intl., Inc.
    P.O. Box 2
    Wilmot, WI 53192

Bedoukian Research Inc.
    Finance Drive
    Danbury, CT 06810
Bell Flavors & Fragrances, Inc.
    500 Academy Drive
    Northbrook, IL 60062
Belle-Aire Fragrances, Inc.
    1500 Old Deerfield Rd.
    Highland Park, IL 60035
Belmay Co.
    35-02 48th Ave.
    Long Island City, NY 11101
Berje, Inc.
    5 Lawrence St.
    Bloomfield, NJ 07003
Brown & Sons, Inc.
    118 S. Center St.
    Bremen, IN 46506
Bush Boake Allen, Inc.
    7 Mercedes Dr.
    Montvale, NJ 07645

Camilli, Albert, & Laloue
    230 Brighton Rd.
    Clifton, NJ 07012
Caswell-Massey (Catalog)
    111 Eighth Ave.
    New York, NY 10011
Centerchem, Inc.
    475 Park Ave. S.
    New York, NY 10016

Centflor Mfg. Co.
    545 W. 45th St.
    New York, NY 10036
Charabot & Co.
    83 Cedar Lane
    Englewood, NJ 07631
Chem-FLeur, Inc.
    200 Pulaski St.
    Newark, NJ 07105
Chemical Dynamics Corp.
    3001 Hadley Rd.
    S. Plainfield, NJ 07080
Citrus & Allied Essences, Ltd.
    65 S. Tyson Ave.
    Floral Park, NY 11001
Compagnie Parento, Inc.
    Westerly Rd.
    Ossining, NY 10562
Creations Aeromatics
    62-12 32nd Ave.
    Woodside, NY 11377
Creative Fragrances Mfg., Inc.
    10420 Plano Rd.
    Dallas, TX 75238
Creative Perfumers
    40 Broad St.
    Carlstadt, NJ 07072

Desmo Chemical Corp.
    8 Westchester Plaza
    Elmsford, NY 10523
Dominion Products, Inc.
    882 Third Ave.
    Brooklyn, NY 11232

Elias Fragrances, Inc.
    999 E. 46th St.
    Brooklyn, NY 11203
Emery Industries
    1300 Carew Tower
    Cincinnati, OH 45202
The Essential Oil Co.
    P.O. Box 88
    Sandy, OR 97055

Felton International, Inc.
    599 Johnson Ave.
    Brooklyn, NY 11237
Firmenich, Inc.
    P.O. Box 5880
    Princeton, NJ 08540
Florasynth, Inc.
    410 E. 62nd St.
    New York, NY 10021

SUPPLIERS

Floressence Parfums Oils, Inc.
21 South Mall
Plainview, NY 11803

Fragrance of the Soul
85-45 151 St.
Jamaica, NY 11431

Fritzche Dodge & Olcott, Inc.
76 Ninth Ave.
New York, NY 10011

Frontier Cooperative Herbs
Box 299
Norway, IA 52318

G's Herbs Intl.
2344 NW 21st Pl.
Portland, OR 97210

Givaudan Corp.
100 Delawanna Ave.
Clifton, NJ 07014

Greef & Co.
1445 E. Putnam Ave.
Old Greenwich, CT 06870

Indiana Botanic Gardens, Inc.
626 177th St.
P.O. Box 5
Hammond, IN 46325

Ingredient Technology Corp.
10 Pelham Pkwy.
Pelham Manor, NY 10803

International Flavors & Fragrances, Inc.
1515 Hwy. #36
Union Beach, NJ 07735

Ivolin Enterprises
500 Fifth Ave.
New York, NY 10110-0395

JPM Imports
48-10 Astoria Blvd.
Astoria, NY 11103

Kalamazoo Spice Extraction Co.
P.O. Box 511
Kalamazoo, MI 49005

Lebermuth Co.
P.O. Box 4103
South Bend, IN 46634

Dr. Madis Laboratories, Inc.
375 Huyler St.
South Hackensack, NJ 07606

Mane Fils, Inc.
16 Spielman Rd.
Fairfield, NJ 07006

Manheimer, Inc.
47-22 Pearson Pl.
Long Island City, NY 11101

Meer Corp.
9500 Railroad Ave.
North Bergen, NJ 07047

Naarden Intl. USA, Inc.
919 Third Ave.
New York, NY 10022

Natural Products Supply Co.
24 E. Burd St.
Shippenburg, PA 17257

Neal & Co.
19th & East Franklin Sts.
P.O. Box 24
Richmond, VA 23201

Nickstadt-Moeller, Inc.
P.O. Box 6
North Bergen, NJ 07047

Norda (Division of PPF)
140 Route 10
East Hanover, NJ 07936

Northville Laboratories, Inc.
P.O. Box 190
One Vanilla Lane
Northville, MI 48167

Noville Essential Oil Co.
1312 Fifth St.
North Bergen, NJ 07047

Nu Essence
P.O. Box 738
Seattle, WA 98111

Penick Corp.
1050 Wall St. W.
Lyndhurst, NJ 07071

Penta Mfg. Co.
P.O. Box 1452
West Caldwell, NJ 07007

Pfaltz & Bauer, Inc.
375 Fairfield Ave.
Stamford, CT 06902

PFW Div. Hercules, Inc.
33 Sprague Ave.
Middletown, NY 10940

Polarome Mfg. Co.
22 Ericsson Place
New York, NY 10013

PPF International
50 Williams Dr.
Ramsey, NJ 07446

Quintessence, Inc.
9002 Chancellor Row
Dallas, TX 75247

Ra-Bob Intl.
320 Hillsdale Dr.
Wichita, KS 67230

Reynaud Ltd.
10 Plant Rd.
Hasbrouck Heights, NJ 07604

Ritter, F. & Co.
    4001 Goodwin Ave.
    P.O. Box 39696
    Los Angeles, CA 90039
Robertet, Inc.
    125 Bauer Dr.
    Oakland, NJ 07436-3190
Roure Bertrand Dupont Inc.
    1775 Windsor Rd.
    Teaneck, NJ 07666

SCM Organic Chemicals-Aroma & Flavor
    P.O. Box 389
    Jacksonville, FL 32201
Shaw Mudge & Co.
    16 Dyke Lane
    Stamford, CT 06902
SITCO
    360 Georges Rd.
    North Brunswick, NJ 08902
The Soap Opera
    319 State St.
    Madison, WI 53703
Star & Crescent Herbs
    8561 Thys Ct.
    Sacramento, CA 95828
Stellar Visions
    808 Post St. #93
    San Francisco, CA 94109
Sunshine Oils
    1919 S. Burnside Ave.
    Los Angeles, CA 90016
Synarome Corp. of America
    55 Vandam St.
    New York, NY 10013
Synfleur
    585 Winters Ave.
    Paramus, NJ 07652

Takasago Corp. USA
    100 Green St.
    Teterboro, NJ 07608

Uncommon Scents
    555 High St.
    Eugene, OR 97401
Ungerer & Co.
    4 Bridgewater Lane
    P.O. Box U
    Lincoln Park, NJ 07035
Universal Fragrance Corp.
    124 Case Dr.
    South Plainfield, NJ 07080
Universal Preserva-Chem, Inc.
    284 North Sixth St.
    Brooklyn, NY 11211
UOP Fragrances US
    43-23 37th Ave.
    Long Island City, NY 11101

Virginia Dare Extract Co.
    882 Third Ave.
    Brooklyn, NY 11232

The Whole Herb Co.
    (Agents for Berje)
    P.O. Box 1085
    Mill Valley, CA 94942

CANADIAN

Bush, Boake, Allen Co. Ltd.
    312 St. Patrick
    La Salle 660
    Montreal, Quebec

Felton International Inc.
    601 Garyray Drive
    Weston, Ontario
Firmenich of Canada Ltd.
    30 Finley
    Bramalea, Ontario
Florasynth Canada Limited
    989 Cote Street
    Montreal, 128, Quebec
Fritzsche, Dodge and Olcott Canada Ltd.
    81 Northline Road
    Toronto 37Y, Ontario

Givaudan (Canada) Ltd.
    60 Overlea
    Toronto, Ontario
Griffiths Laboratories Ltd.
    757 Pharmacy Ave.
    Scarborough, Ontario

Haarman and Reimer
    1355 Aerowood Drive
    Toronto, Ontario

International Flavors and Fragrances Ltd.
    7330 Keele Street N.
    Concord, Ontario

R.W. Love Ltd.
    39 Parliament Street
    Toronto, Ontario

Norda Ltd.
    833 King Street West
    Toronto, Ontario

Stange Canada Ltd.
    3340 Orlando Drive
    Malton, Ontario
Stuart Brothers, Division of Givaudan Ltd.
    3470 St. Antoine Street
    Montreal, Quebec

FRANCE

Alphonse Isnard
    36, rue Jules Massenet
    94 Vincennes

Bertrand Frères
    Avenue Font-Laugiere
    06 Grasse

Bruno Court-S.A. Jean Roure
    P.O. Box 58
    06 Grasse

Camilli Albert et Laloue
    27, avenue Sainte-Lorette
    06 Grasse

Descollonges Frères SA
    13, rue du Canada
    69 Villeurbanne

Ets. Charabot et Cie
    83 Seillans

Ets. Laserson et Sabetay
    14, rue Jean Ronal
    92 La Garenne-Colombes

Fabriques de Laire
    129, quai de Stalingrad
    92 Issy-les-Moulineaux

Givaudan S.a.r.l. Division
    Esrolko
    48, avenue Pierre-Curie
    78 Le Pecq

H. Reynaud et Fils
    26570 Montbrun Les Bains

International Flavours and Fragrances (IFF)
    France S.a.r.l.
    47, rue Victor Hugo
    92 Bois-Colombes

Isnard-Maubert SA
    Avenue Pierre-Semard
    06 Grasse

Lautier Fils
    Avenue Fort-Laugiere
    06 Grasse

Marcel Vian
    06 Golfe-Juan

Mero et Boyeau
    Benard et Honnorat
    55, bd. Victor Hugo
    06 Grasse

Parfumerie Jean Niel
    4, rue Tracastel
    06 Grasse

Payan et Bertrand
    Avenue Jean XXIII
    06 Grasse

Roure Bertrand Fils et Justin Dupont
    27, avenue Pierre Semard
    06 Grasse

S.A. Tombarel Frères
    7, avenue Pierre Samard
    06 Grasse

Sté Chrysa
    69 Fontaines s/Saone

Sté D. Blayn et Cie
    60, avenue du General Leclerc
    94 Maisons-Alfort

Sté Givaudan France
    44, bd. du Parc
    92 Neuilly s/Saine

Sté Firmenich et Cie
    93, avenue de Neuilly
    92 Neuilly s/Seine

Sté Naarden (France)
    82, rue P.V. Couturier
    92 Levallois-Perret

U.O.P. Fragrances (de Trevise)
    42-48, rue de la Reine Henrietta
    92 Colombes

U.O.P Fragrances (formerly A. Chiris)
    Avenue Pierre Semard
    06 Grasse

V. Mane Fils
    06 Bar-sur-Loup

Other Useful Addresses in France

Central Essential Oils & Aromatic Raw Materials Assn.
*Syndicat Dentral des Huiles Essentialles et Matières
    Premières Aromatiques*
    2, rue de Penthievre
    Paris 8e

Association of Grasse Brokers
Syndicat des Courtiers Grassois
    c/o C.C. Leroux
    Villa Chanteclerc

Manufacturers and Importers of Essential Oils
*Syndicat National des Fabricants et Importateurs d'Huiles
    Essentielles et Produits Aromatiques Naturels*
    7, rue Gazan
    Grasse

National Assn. of Mfg. of Synthetic Aromatic Products
*Syndicat National des Fabricants de Produits Aromatiques
    de Synthese*
    57, avenue Marceau
    Paris 16 e

UNITED KINGDOM

Fragrance Houses

Bush Boake Allen
    Blackhorse Lane
    Walthamshire, London E17 SQP

Clayton & Jowett Ltd.
    Runcorn WA 7 1PJ

Firmenich Co.
    Hayes Road
    Southall
    Middlesex

Fritzsche, Dodge and Olcott (UK) Ltd.
    Finedon Road Industrial Estate
    Links Road
    Wellingborough, Northants

Fuerst Day, Lawson Ltd.
    St. Clare House
    30-33 Minores
    London EC3N 1LN

Givaudan and Co., Ltd.
    Godstone Road
    Whyteleafe, Surrey

IFF (Great Britain) Ltd.
    Crown Road
    Enfield, Middlesex

Lautier Fils Ltd.
    Power Rd.
    London W4

Lionel Hitchens (Essential Oils) Ltd.
    50 Albert Road North
    Reigate, Surrey

Lofil Ltd.
    Power Road
    London W4

Naarden (London) Ltd.
    73 Upper Richmond Rd.
    London SW15

Norda International Ltd.
    Stirling Road
    Slough SL1 4TA

Oxford Chemicals Ltd.
    Shires Road
    Brackley, Northamptonshire NN13 5EZ

Proprietary Perfumes Ltd.
    Ashford, Kent

UOP Fragrances Ltd.
    39 East Cheap
    Epsom, Surrey

Distributors

W.H. Hobbs and Co. Ltd.
    166 Tower Bridge Road
    London SE1

R.C. Treatt and Co. Ltd.
    Northern Way
    Bury St. Edmunds
    Suffolk IP32 6NL

GERMANY

Most are members of the Verband der Deutschen Essenzenindutrie, E.V. (Association of the German Fragrance and Flavor Industry, Inc.) Neusserstrasse 104, 5000 Cologne. Ask them for a current list.

Andreas Horlin und Co. KG
    Am Kreuzstein 7-9
    8650 Kulbach

Deutsche "Naarden" GmbH
    P.O. Box 660160
    2 Hamburg 66

Erich Ziegler, Aroma Chemie
    Haus Nr. 143
    Aufsess 8551

Ewald Reichel
    Grossbeerenstrasse 9-11
    1000 Berlin 42

Fritzche Dodge und Olcott GmbH
    Allensteiner Strasse 2
    4970 Bad Oeynhausen

Gelsenberg-Chemie GmbH
    Rosastrasse 2
    4300 Easen

Gerberding und Co.—Dragoco
    Spezialfabrik kinzentrierter Riech—und
    Aromastoffe
    Dragocostrasse
    3450 Holzminden

Givaudan GmbH
    Gutenbergring 2-6
    2 Norderstedt 3

Grau Aromatics
    7070 Schwabisch Gmund
    West Germany

Haarman und Reimer GmbH
    An den Teichen 2
    3450 Holzminden

Henkel KGaA
    ZR-KH Aromatic Chemicals
    P.O. Box 1100—4000 Dusseldorf 1
    West Germany

International Flavors & Fragrances IFF
(Deutschland) GmbH
4240 Emmerich

Johannes Vogele KG
Bahnhofatstrasse 143
7128 Lauffen

Otto Reichel
Elbestrasse 28-29
1000 Berlin 44

Schimmel und Co. GmbH (Norda affiliate)
Billbrookdeich
200 Hamburg 74

UOP Fragrances GmbH
Försterweg 81
1000 Hamburg 54

Westfalische Essenzenfabrik
Von der Tannstrasse
4600 Dortmund

JAPAN

Japan Flavour and Fragrance Manufacturer's Assn.
Nomura Bldg., 3rd Floor
No 2, 3-chome
Kodenmacho, Nihonbashi
Chuo-ku, Tokyo

Ogawa and Co. Ltd.
3-3 Hirano-cho,
Higashi-ku, Tokyo

San-ei Chemical Industries Ltd.
1-1, Sanwa-cho
Toyonaka City, Osaka

Shiono Koryo Kaisha Ltd.
No 3-11 Doshomachi
Higashi-ku, Osaka

Soda Aromatic Co. Ltd.
4-14- Honcho
Nihonbashi
Chuo-ku, Tokyo

Takasago Perfumery Co. Ltd.
1-4-1, Hatchobori
Chuo-ki, Tokyo

Tanemura & Co. Ltd.
P.O. Box 969
Central Tokyo, 10091

Toyotama Perfumery Co. Ltd.
1-5 Honcho, Nihonbashi
Chuo-ku, Tokyo

POLAND

Inter-Fragrances
P.O. Box 45
Poznan
(Importer of aromatic raw materials and essential oils for Eastern European countries)

EGYPT

N.I. Ibrahim Co.
8, Falaki St.
Alexandria
(Egyptian natural essential oils, botanicals, spices, and herbs: geranium, cumin, basil, jasmine, cassie, concretes, and more)

INDIA

Synthite-Industrial Chemicals Private Ltd.
Ajay Vihar
M.G. Road
Cochin—682 016
(Superb quality spice oils, oleoresins, and food colors)

TURKEY

Konurlar S.A.
Boite Postale 79
Mecidiyekov
Istanbul
(Rose oil supplier)

BIBLIOGRAPHY

Arctander, Steffan, *Perfume and Flavor Materials of Natural Origin*, Elizabeth, N.J.: self-published, 1960.

Arctander, Steffan, *Perfume and Flavor Chemicals*, Elizabeth, N.J.: self published.

Bailes, Edith G., *An Album of Fragrance*, Richmond, Me. Cardamom, 1983.

Bedoukian, Dr. Paul, *Perfumery and Flavor Materials*, Wheaton, Ill.: Allured Pub., (no date). *Perfumer and Flavorist Magazine* compilation of 38 years of annual review articles on development of perfumery, flavoring, and essential oils.

Bernard, Bruce K. (ed.), *Flavor and Fragrance Materials 1985*, Wheaton, Ill.: Allured Pub., 1985.

Clifford, F. S., *Romance of Perfume*, New York: Gordon Press, 1977.

Conway, David, *Magic: An Occult Primer*, New York: Bantam, 1972.

Cooley, Arnold J., *The Toilet and Cosmetic Arts in Ancient and Modern Times*, Franklin, (1866) 1970.

Crowley, Aleister, *The Qabala of Aleister Crowley*, New York: Samuel Weiser, 1973.

Crowley, Aleister, *Magick in Theory and Practice*, New York: Castle Books, (no date).

Cunningham-Carter, Lady Sara, *The Arts Magian*, Glendale, Ore.: privately published, 1974.

Denning and Phillips, *Magical States of Consciousness*, St. Paul: Llewellyn Pubns, 1985.

Firth, Grace, *Secrets of the Still*, McLean, Va.: EPM Pubns, 1983.

Gaborit, Jean-Yves, *Perfumes: The Essence and Their Bottles*, New York: Rizzoli Intl. Pub. Inc., 1985.

Gattefosse, R. M., *Formulary of Perfumery*, London, 1952.

Genders, Roy, *Perfume through the Ages*, New York: G.P. Putnam's Sons, 1972.

Genders, Roy, *Perfume in the Garden*, London: Museum Press, 1955.

Guenther, E., *The Essential Oils*, vol. I–VI, Huntington, New York: Robt. E. Krieger, 1972.

Hall, R. D., Klemme, D., and Nienhaus, J., *The H & R Book. Guide to Fragrance Ingredients*, London: Johnson Pub., 1985.

Hand, Robert, *Horoscope Symbols*, Rockport, Mass.: Para Research, 1981.

Hamaker-Zondag, Dr. Karen, *Planetary Symbolism in the Horoscope*, vol. 2, New York: Samuel Weiser, 1985.

Jellinek, Paul, *The Practice of Modern Perfumery*, London, 1954.

Jessee, Jill, *Perfume Album*, Huntington, N.Y.: Kreiger, 1965 (1974).

Junius, Manfred M., *The Practical Handbook of Plant Alchemy*, Rochester, Vt.: Inner Traditions, 1985.

Kaufman, William I., *Perfume*, New York: E.P. Dutton, 1974.

de Laurence, L. W., *The Greater Key of Solomon*, Chicago, Ill.: de Laurence, Scott and Co., 1914.

Lawrence, Dr. Brian M., *Essential Oils, 1976–1978*, Wheaton, Ill.: Allured, 1978.

Leek, Sybil, *Sybil Leek's Astrological Guide to Successful Everyday Living*, New York: New American Library, 1972.

Levi, Eliphas, *Transcendental Magic*, New York: Samuel Weiser, 1970.

Maple, Eric, *The Magic of Perfume*, New York: Samuel Weiser, 1973.

Maurer, Edward S., *Perfumes and their Production*, London: United Trade Press, Ltd., 1958.

McKenzie, Dr. D., *Aromatics and the Soul*.

Miller, Richard, *The Magical and Ritual Use of Herbs*, Rochester, Vt.: Inner Traditions, 1983.

Miller, Richard, *The Magical and Ritual Use of Aphrodisiacs*, Rochester, Vt.: Inner Traditions, 1985.

Moldenke, Harold and Alma, *Plants of the Bible*, New York: Dover, 1986.

Morris, Edwin T., *Fragrance: The Story of Perfume from Cleopatra to Chanel*, New York: Scribner, 1985.

Morrison, Sarah, *The Modern Witch's Spellbook*, vol. I–II, Citadel Pr.: Secaucus, N.J., 1973, 1986.

Mueller, Arno, *Internationaler Riechstoff Kodex*, Heuthig, 1968.

Muller, J., *The H & R Book of Perfume. Understanding Fragrance: Origin, History, Development, and Meaning*, London: Johnson Pub., 1984.

Muller, J., *The H & R Book Fragrance Guide: Feminine Notes*, London: Johnson Pub., 1984.

Muller, J., *The H & R Book Fragrance Guide: Masculine Notes*, London: Johnson Pub., 1985.

Parry, E. J., *Cyclopedia of Perfumery*.

Pelton, Robert W., *The Complete Book of Voodoo*, New York: Berkeley Medallion, 1972.

Piesse, Charles H., *The Art of Perfumery*, London: Piesse & Lubin, 1891.

Plummer, Beverly, *Fragrance*, New York: Atheneum, 1975.

Porta, John Baptista, *Natural Magick*, New York: Basic Books, 1957.

Poucher, W. A. and Howard, G. M., *Perfumes, Cosmetics and Soaps*, vol. I–III, London: Chapman & Hall, Methuen, 1975.

Poucher, P. W., *Journal of the Society of Cosmetic Chemists*, vol. VI, 1955.

Pownall, G., *Perfumery*, Wellington, England: Seven Seas Pub., 1974.

Regardie, Israel, *The Middle Pillar*, St. Paul, Minn.: Llewellyn Pub., 1970.

Regardie, Israel, *The Tree of Life*, New York: Samuel Weiser, 1969.

Rimmel, Eugene, *The Book of Perfumes*.

Rohde, Eleanor Sinclair, *Rose Recipes from Olden Times*, New York: Dover, 1973.

Rovesti, P., *In Search of Perfumes Lost*, Venice: Blow Up, 1980.

Sagarin, Edward S., *The Science and Art of Perfumery*, New York: Greenberg, 1955.

Santin de Riols, E.-N., *Les Parfums Magiques* (Magic Perfumes), Paris: Library Francaise, L. Genoceaux & Cie, ed., 1903.

Shelmerdine, Cynthia W., *The Perfume Industry of Mycenaean Pylos*, Gateborg, Ger.: Paul Astrome Forlag, 1985.

Stone, Philo (Richard and Iona Miller), *Pantheon: Gods and Goddesses in Daily Life*, unpublished.

———, *The Holistic Qabala*, unpublished.

Theimer, Ernst T., *Fragrance Chemistry: The Science of the Sense of Smell*, New York: Academic Press, 1982.

Tisserand, Robert, *The Art of Aromatherapy*, Rochester, Vt.: Healing Arts Press, 1977.

Thompson, C. J. S., *The Mystery and Lure of Perfume*, London: John Lane the Bodley Head Ltd., 1927.

Trueman, J., *The Romantic Story of Scent*, Garden City, N.Y.: Doubleday, 1975.

Valnet, Jean, *The Practice of Aromatherapy*, Rochester, Vt.: Healing Arts Press, 1982.

Wang, Robert, *The Qabalistic Tarot*, York Beach, Me.: Samuel Weiser, 1983.

Wells, F. V. and Billot, Marcel, *Perfumery Technology: Art, Science and Technology*, 2nd ed., New York: Halstead, 1981.

Winter, Ruth, *The Smell Book*, Philadelphia: J.B. Lippincott Co., 1976.

APPENDIX

Correspondence Reference Guide

KEY	HEBREW/ENGLISH	ASTROLOGY	NAME	TONE	COLOR	SCENTS
Essence of the Spheres						
1		Origin	Kether		White	Ambergris
2		Zodiac	Chokmah		Gray	Musk
3		Saturn	Binah		Black	Myrrh, civet, madonna lily
4		Jupiter	Chesed		Blue	Cedar, oakmoss
5		Mars	Geburah		Red	Tobacco, leather
6		Sun	Tiphareth		Yellow	Olibanum (frankincense), angelica
7		Venus	Netzach		Green	Benzoin, rose, sandalwood
8		Mercury	Hod		Orange	Storax, amber, spikenard
9		Moon	Yesod		Violet	Jasmine, ginseng, orris
10		Earth	Malkuth		Tertiaries	Dittany of Crete, poppy, patchouli
Essence of the Paths						
11	א/A	Air	Fool	E	Yellow	Galbanum
12	ב/B	Mercury	Magician	E	Orange	Storax, mastic
13	ג/G	Moon	Priestess	G#	Violet	Camphor, aloes
14	ד/D	Venus	Empress	F#	Green	Sandalwood, myrtle
15	ה/H	Aries	Emperor	C	Scarlet	Dragon's blood
16	ו/V	Taurus	Hierophant	C#	Red-Orange	Storax
17	ז/Z	Gemini	Lovers	D	Orange	Wormwood, orchid
18	ח/Ch	Cancer	Chariot	D#	Orange-Yellow	Onycha, lotus, labdanum
19	ט/T	Leo	Strength	E#	Yellow	Olibanum (frankincense)
20	י/Y,I	Virgo	Hermit	F	Yellow-Green	Narcissus
21	כ/K	Jupiter	Wh. of Fortune	A#	Blue	Saffron
22	ל/L	Libra	Adjustment	F#	Green	Galbanum
23	מ/M	Water	Hanged Man	G#	Blue	Onycha, myrrh
24	נ/N	Scorpio	Death	G	Blue-Green	Benzoin, opopanax
25	ס/S	Sagittarius	Art	G#	Blue	Lign-aloes
26	ע/O	Capricorn	The Devil	A	Violet	Musk, civet
27	פ/P	Mars	Tower	C	Red	Pepper, dragon's blood
28	צ/Tz	Aquarius	The Star	A#	Purple	Galbanum
29	ק/Q	Pisces	The Moon	B	Magenta	Ambergris, lily, honeysuckle, violet
30	ר/R	Sun	The Sun	D	Yellow	Olibanum, cinnamon
31	ש/Sh	Fire	The Aeon	C	Red	Olibanum
32	ת/T	Saturn	Universe	A	Indigo	Storax, castoreum, cypress

= sharp note

INGREDIENT INDEX

acacia, 23, 24, 57, 96, 125, 126
agar oil, 106, 146
allspice, 121, 142
aloe vera, 130
aloe-wood (see agar oil), 5, 33, 65, 70, 85, 106, 120, 121, 122, 146
almond, 18, 22, 23, 24, 138
amaryllis, 130
amber aldehyde, 38
amber oil, 32, 33, 49, 56, 57, 60, 67, 120, 133, 134, 139, 142, 150, 152, 153, 155
ambergris, 18, 19, 20, 23, 24, 26, 28, 33, 36–39, 41, 42, 63, 64, 65, 70, 95, 106, 111, 115, 120, 121, 146, 155, 157
ambrette seed oil, 18, 23, 28, 42, 152
ammoniacum, 142
amyris, 18, 27, 138
angelica oil, 18, 27, 28, 29, 33, 42, 92, 96, 126
anise, 18, 26, 92, 101, 111, 121, 133, 138, 142
apple blossom, 70, 126
araucaria, 146
arnica, 141, 142
artemesia, 138
atractylis, 152
asafetida, 28, 115, 121, 142
azalea, 96, 126

balm melissa, 23, 142
balsams, 25
barberry, 141, 142
basil oil, 18, 28, 52, 88, 90, 118, 121, 142
bayberry, 121, 122
bay oil, 2, 18, 88, 92, 93, 96, 107, 121, 126, 146
begonia, 157
benzaldehyde, 43, 138
benzene, 14, 47, 60, 69, 78
benzoic acid, 64
benzoin oil (benjamin), 23, 24, 27, 28, 32, 33, 38, 46, 56, 62–64, 70, 104, 120, 130, 138
bergamot oil, 18, 23, 24, 25, 28, 29, 56, 57, 60, 66, 67, 77, 88, 90, 95, 98, 105, 109, 111, 121, 126, 134, 135, 138, 139, 142, 143, 146, 149, 150, 152
birch tar oil, 18, 56, 57, 118, 121, 138
bois de rose (see rose), 18, 28, 52, 142
bois de siam, 138
boronia, 52, 111, 150, 155
bouvardia, 157
broom oil, 134
buchu, 146

cactus flower 142
cajeput, 18
calamus oil, 18, 24, 46, 52, 65, 84, 95, 121, 135, 142, 150
camellia, 74, 137, 138

camphor oil, 5, 18, 23, 24, 29, 33, 43, 85–86, 120, 121, 122, 130
Canada balsam, 146
cananga, 18, 28, 56, 130, 150, 152
canella, 142
caraway, 23
cardomom, 18, 121, 134, 138
carnation oil, 14, 18, 19, 23, 28, 66, 70, 98, 108, 122, 134, 135, 142, 146
carrot seed, 18, 134
cascarilla, 18, 146
cassia oil, 18, 23, 28, 46, 66, 67, 70, 78, 96, 122, 126, 134, 155
cassie oil, 14, 18, 23, 52, 155
castoreum, 33, 56, 133, 134, 143, 146, 150, 152
cedarwood oil, 18, 23, 25, 28, 33, 50–53, 56, 67, 78, 92, 100, 106, 121, 122, 127, 134, 135, 138, 142, 143, 145, 146, 150
celery oil, 130
chamomile, 18, 28, 95, 96, 115, 126, 150, 155
champaca, 134
chaulmoogra oil, 39, 42
cinnamic alcohol, 52, 61, 64, 70, 71, 78, 82, 98, 107, 126, 130, 134, 150, 152
cinnamon oil, 2, 18, 23, 24, 25, 33, 38, 46, 56, 60, 61, 96, 106, 112, 113, 118, 119, 121, 122, 126, 130, 138, 142
cistus (labdanum) oil, 18, 23, 28, 29, 38, 52, 60, 61, 67, 78, 94–95, 103, 104, 115, 127
citron, 18, 22, 122
citronella, 18, 24, 28, 138
citrus, 13, 29, 74, 84, 90, 95, 107, 110, 126, 127, 134, 135, 138, 139, 142, 146, 150, 152, 153, 155
civet, 18, 20, 23, 24, 25, 26, 27, 28, 33, 38, 41, 42, 47–49, 65, 107, 120, 121, 134, 149
clematis, 22
clove oil, 18, 23, 24, 28, 56, 67, 70, 78, 89, 98, 100, 111, 120, 121, 122, 126, 134, 135, 142, 146, 150
clover oil, 19, 43, 66, 146, 152
coriander, 18, 23, 28, 90, 105, 118, 121, 134, 138, 142
costus oil, 18, 28, 39, 66, 67, 135, 142, 150, 155
coumarin, 28, 29, 49, 57, 61, 70, 78, 126, 134, 135, 138, 142, 146, 150, 153, 155
cucumber, 130
cumin, 18, 28, 101, 138
cyclamen, 70, 138, 152
cyperus oil, 134, 155
cypress oil, 18, 28, 33, 39, 47, 52, 70, 102, 107, 115, 121, 122, 130, 138, 150

datura oil, 150, 157
davana, 146

dill oil, 18, 23, 84, 106, 118, 121
dittany of Crete, 33, 77
dargon's blood, 33

elecampane, 130, 152
elemi, 18, 28, 108, 130, 139, 152
eucalyptus, 18, 25, 86, 96, 121, 125, 126
eugenol (clove), 20, 45, 66, 67, 98, 108, 142
everlasting, 27, 146

fennel, 18, 23, 118, 121, 134
fenugreek, 134
fern, 29, 52, 64, 70, 78, 82, 84, 95, 134, 138, 146, 155
fir, 105, 130, 146
fougere (see fern)
frangipani, 24, 74, 130
frankincense (see olibanum) xii, 2, 15, 28, 31, 52, 53, 58–61, 94, 96, 119, 122, 125, 126
freesia, 138

galangal, 96, 113, 121, 126
galbanum, 18, 24, 28, 33, 81–82, 94, 101, 102, 109, 118, 121, 134, 138
gardenia, 19, 20, 82, 110, 129, 130, 138, 150
geraniol, 67, 107, 155
geranium, 13, 18, 23, 24, 25, 28, 47, 66, 67, 78, 102, 121, 134, 142, 146
ginger, 18, 28, 121, 135, 142, 152
ginseng, 33, 130
grains of paradise, 120, 126
guaiac wood, 18, 28, 53, 66

heather, 134
helichrysum, 155
heliotrope, 14, 19, 22, 24, 96, 125, 126, 130, 139
honey, 142
honeysuckle, 33, 83, 122, 126, 130, 134
hyacinth, 18, 19, 23, 70, 82, 93, 97, 134, 135, 143
hyssop, 88, 106, 121, 146

ionones, 20, 52, 61, 67, 78, 98, 111, 126, 130, 133, 134, 135, 138, 139, 142, 150, 152, 155
iris (see orris), 28
isoeugenol, 20, 28, 82, 90, 108, 130, 131, 134, 138, 152, 155

jasmine, 5, 14, 18, 19, 20, 23, 24, 25, 28, 33, 38, 56, 57, 64, 65, 66, 70, 72–75, 93, 95, 98, 102, 118, 121, 122, 129, 130, 131, 134, 135, 138, 142, 143, 150, 155
jonquil, 14, 18, 20, 23, 24, 70
juniper berry, 18, 25, 28, 47, 67, 130, 146, 150, 153

167

labdanum (see cistus), 28, 29, 33, 38, 39, 52, 56, 57, 78, 94–95, 105, 115, 130, 133, 134, 138, 139, 142, 143, 150, 152, 153, 155, 157
laurel, 18, 23, 146
lavender oil, 13, 18, 19, 23, 24, 25, 26, 38, 56, 57, 67, 70, 78, 82, 83, 84, 88, 92, 93, 95, 102, 107, 109, 110, 115, 118, 121, 126, 127, 130, 134, 135, 138, 139, 146, 150, 152, 153, 155
lavendin, 86, 88, 95, 107, 130, 138
leather, 29, 33, 135, 142, 152
lemon, 18, 22, 23, 25, 26, 38, 95, 118, 121
lemongrass, 18, 126
lign-aloes, 33, 106
lilac, 19, 20, 70, 74, 130, 134, 135, 146
lily of the valley, 14, 19, 20, 23, 28, 33, 43, 49, 56, 61, 70, 74, 97, 110, 120, 126, 130, 134, 138, 142, 146, 150
lime, 18, 23, 88, 90, 133, 134, 142
linalool, 18, 28, 47, 67, 70, 82, 89, 106, 126, 130, 131, 134, 138, 146, 150
liquidamber, 39, 68, 69
lotus, 33, 94, 126, 130
lovage, 18, 104, 130, 138

mace, 23, 120, 121, 122
madonna lily, 33, 45, 148
magnolia, 24, 149, 150
marigold, 2, 96, 125, 126
marjoram, 18, 23, 25, 28, 70, 92, 120, 134
mastic, 18, 28, 33, 83, 84, 92, 93, 98, 118, 121, 122, 130, 135
mignonette, 23, 146
mimosa, 14, 18, 19, 28, 52, 61, 65, 66, 67, 70, 83, 98, 105, 111, 130, 134, 138, 155
mint (see spearmint & peppermint), 101
monarda, 146
muguet (see lily of the valley)
musks, 10, 18, 19, 23, 24, 25, 26, 27, 28, 29, 33, 38, 40, 41–43, 49, 57, 64, 65, 67, 70, 105, 107, 115, 121, 122, 134, 138, 139, 142, 153, also nitro musk
myrrh oil, 18, 24, 28, 33, 44–47, 59, 78, 81, 103, 104, 106, 120, 121, 125, 149 150
myrtle oil, 28, 33, 87, 91, 120, 121, 122, 126, 140
myrtlewood oil, 107

narcissus, 18, 23, 33, 49, 70, 82, 97–98, 100, 120, 134, 135, 137, 138, 146, 157
narde (see spikenard)
neroli, 13, 18, 19, 23, 24, 25, 26, 29, 56, 57, 74, 78, 100, 105, 127, 131, 135, 138, 139, 150, 152, 155

new mown hay, 24, 64, 134
nitro musk, 47, 49, 52, 61, 78, 95, 105, 127, 130, 139, 142, 150, 152, 153
nutmeg, 18, 23, 28, 70, 96, 100, 121, 122, 146

oakmoss, 14, 23, 27, 28, 29, 33, 39, 57, 67, 78, 82, 90, 93, 95, 126, 130, 134, 135, 138, 139, 142, 143, 146, 150, 153, 155
olibanum (see frankincense), 18, 24, 27, 28, 29, 33, 39, 52, 57, 58–61, 94, 96, 98, 112, 113, 114, 118, 121, 126, 127, 138, 139, 142, 157
onycha (see labdanum)
opopanax, 18, 28, 45, 67, 78, 90, 91, 95, 104, 126, 130, 135, 138, 139, 142, 150, 152
orange oil, sweet, 24, 134
orange, 14, 18, 22, 23, 24, 38, 49, 61, 66, 70, 93, 98, 130, 131, 138, 143
orange, mandarin, 18, 47
orchid, 33, 91, 92, 135, 138
origanum, 18, 28, 90, 127
orris root oil, 18, 23, 24, 28, 29, 33, 42, 65, 70, 78, 121, 135, 138, 152, 155

palmarosa, 18
passionflower, 96, 126
patchouli, 10, 18, 20, 23, 24, 25, 27, 28, 29, 33, 38, 39, 47, 52, 53, 57, 64, 66, 67, 76, 77, 78, 91, 105, 121, 126, 130, 134, 135, 138, 139, 142, 146, 150, 153
peony, 96, 127
pepper, black, 33, 108, 146
peppermint, 18, 23, 24, 29, 101, 138
pergalaria, 24
Peru balsam, 18, 23, 24, 28, 29, 39, 66, 146, 147
petroleum ether, 14, 23, 47
pine, 18, 29, 47, 52, 78, 81, 82, 90, 95, 105, 109, 111, 121, 122, 127, 134, 135, 138, 142, 146, 150, 153
petitgrain, 18, 24, 29, 57, 107, 130

reseda, 14, 18
rhodinol, 134, 142
rose absolute, 66
rose, 12, 14, 18, 19, 20, 22, 23, 24, 25, 26, 28, 32, 33, 38, 43, 49, 52, 56, 57, 62, 63, 64, 65, 67, 70, 78, 88, 87, 98, 108, 118, 120, 121, 122, 126, 134, 135, 137, 138, 142, 146, 150, 152
rose geranium, 64
rose water, 12, 57, 64, 70
rosemary, 18, 23, 25, 85, 88, 96, 107, 109, 122, 126, 127, 134, 138, 142, 146
rue, 18, 23, 120, 127, 153

saffron, 28, 33, 41, 46, 96, 99, 119, 120, 122, 127

sage, 18, 23, 52, 66, 126, 138, 146, 147
sage, clary, 18, 29, 38, 39, 52, 56, 57, 78, 86, 88, 90, 95, 105, 109, 115, 126, 130, 134, 138, 139, 143, 146, 150, 155
sandalwood, 18, 20, 23, 24, 25, 28, 29, 32, 33, 39, 49, 56, 57, 61, 62, 63, 65, 66, 78, 87, 91, 106, 111, 119, 120, 121, 122, 134, 135, 137, 138, 142, 143, 146, 150, 152
sassafras, 18, 28, 52, 53, 138
skatole, 28, 29
snakeroot, Canadian, 142
southernwood, 24
spearmint, 18, 23, 88, 101, 102, 109, 121
spikenard, 28, 32, 33, 95, 118, 121, 135
stock, 14
stephanotis, 130, 157
storax, 23, 24, 28, 29, 32, 33, 38, 56, 64, 69, 70, 82, 83, 91, 115, 120, 130, 133, 134, 135, 138, 139, 146
sumbul, 28, 153
sweet pea, 24, 83, 126, 130
syringa, 23, 24, 153

tangerine, 18
tarragon, 18, 28
thuja, 28, 52
thyme, 28, 86, 88, 126
tobacco, 33, 54, 56, 101, 120, 142, 143
Tolu balsam, 18, 23, 24, 28, 39, 130, 135, 139
tonka bean, 23, 24, 28, 139, 142
tuberose, 14, 18, 23, 24, 67, 70, 74, 98, 130, 131, 134, 135

valerian, 18, 28, 135
vanilla, 22, 23, 24, 28, 42, 49, 91, 121, 126, 130, 135, 142, 150
vanillin, 63, 64, 71, 91
verbena, 18, 19, 22, 24, 28, 56, 95, 118, 152
vetiver, 18, 23, 27, 28, 29, 39, 52, 53, 61, 64, 67, 78, 91, 118, 121, 134, 135, 139, 142, 143, 146, 152
violet, 14, 18, 19, 20, 23, 34, 28, 33, 43, 52, 67, 70, 74, 82, 95, 97, 98, 100, 105, 110, 111, 121, 122, 126, 130, 134, 135, 138, 146, 150, 152

wallflower, 24, 131
wintergreen, 18
wisteria, 135
wormwood, 18, 33, 52, 92–93, 107, 121, 143

ylang-ylang, 18, 19, 25, 28, 52, 70, 73, 98, 107, 111, 121, 126, 130, 131, 134, 135, 138, 146

zedoary (zedoaria), 65

INDEX

abeer (abir), 65, 67
Abramelin (oil of), 34
absinthe, 92, 120
absolute, 23
abyss, 45
active imagination, 7, 79, 80
Adam, 87
Adjustment, 33, 101
The Aeon, 33, 114
Aeone, 116
Air, 33, 81, 117, 118, 119
Ajna chakra, 41
alchemy, xi, 11, 12, 15
aldehydic, 90, 108
Alexander, 65
aloe vera, 106
alpha, 79
altered states of consciousness, 5
Amazon, 63
amber, 91, 95, 108, 115, 134
ambrein, 37, 38
anchor(ing), 4, 5, 7, 8, 10, 34
anima, 73
Anima Mundi, 45
animus, 73
aphrodisiac, 38, 42, 47, 49, 77, 98, 138
Aphrodite, 55, 63, 65, 87, 136–137, 141
Apollo, 31, 59, 107, 124–126, 129
Aquarius, 33, 109, 117, 119, 122
archetypes, 5, 31, 122
Ares, 55, 140, 141
Aries, 33, 89, 117, 121
aromatherapy, 25, 32, 77
Arabia(n), xi, 45, 59, 98, 106
Art, 33, 106
Artemis, 73, 128, 129
Astarte, 137
astral body, 7
astral plane, 5, 6, 119, 121
astral travel, 80, 152
astrology, xi, 80
attar (see otto), 64, 109
Attila, 108
Avicenna, 12, 59, 65

Banishing Ritual, 5, 6, 7, 8, 34, 117, 118
base note, 26, 27, 126, 130, 134, 135, 138, 139, 142, 150, 152, 155
bdellium, 46, 104
Bible, 81
Binah, 33, 44, 45, 103
blotters, 26, 27
bouquet, 16, 17, 18, 95, 98
Britain, 77
Buddha, 59, 67

Caduceus, 133
Cancer, 33, 94, 117, 122
Capricorn, 33, 107, 117, 122
Celts, 111
charkras, 8, 152
The Chariot, 33, 103
chassis, 74

cedrol, 51
Chesed, 33, 50, 51, 53
China, 42, 59, 85, 104, 111, 112
Chokmah, 33, 40, 41, 42
Christ, 2, 46, 59, 60, 125
Chronos, 149, 152
chypre, 29, 47, 52, 63, 66, 69, 78, 82, 90, 93, 95, 105, 110, 126, 134, 142, 146, 150
circle (magic), 6, 7, 117, 118, 122
circulatio, 13
civet cat (*Viverra civetta*), 47
civet-tone, 47
clairvoyance, 80
Cleopatra, 65
coagulatio, 13
collective unconscious, 31
cologne, 17, 25, 28, 88, 95, 110, 122, 126, 127, 134, 142, 146, 152
concrete, 22, 23
coniunctio, 13
consecration, 34
correspondences xi, 1, 4, 31, 32, 79, 117, 118, 121, 157
creativity, 2
Crowley, Aleister, 3, 10, 34, 45, 63, 69, 80, 81, 83, 85, 92, 96, 97, 104, 106, 107, 108, 109, 111, 112, 114, 115, 118, 119
crown-center 8, 37

Daphne, 107
Death, 33, 104
Demeter, 60, 77
The Devil, 107
diamond, xii
Diana, 52, 129
divination, 125
distillation, 11, 12, 13, 26, 65
dreams, 73, 80, 125, 127, 130, 133

earth, 33, 98, 117, 118, 119
eau de cologne, 74, 109
eau de parfum, 17
eau de toilet, 17, 25
ego, 125
Egypt(ians), xi, 45, 59, 65, 83, 95, 125, 133, 146
elixer, 12
Elizabeth I, 91
The Emperor, 33
The Empress, 33
England, 87, 99
enfleurage, 13, 14, 73, 74
Eros, 65
E.S.P. (extrasensory perception), 5
essence, 3, 4, 11, 12, 13, 20, 25, 26, 31, 34, 35, 51, 55, 56, 59, 95, 99
essential oil, 1, 11, 16, 18, 19, 22, 25, 26, 27, 32
Euripedes, 129
expression, 11, 13, 26
extraction, 11, 13, 14, 26, 73

fern (fougere), 29, 52, 64, 70, 78, 82, 102, 105, 106, 110, 126, 134, 135, 142

fire, 12, 33, 96, 108, 114, 117, 118, 119
fixative, 17, 26, 27, 28, 38, 42, 49, 53, 56, 63, 64, 67, 70, 77, 82, 84, 88, 95, 104, 109, 134, 138, 142, 146, 150, 152
floral, 29, 82
The Fool, 33, 81
Fortune, Dion, 80
France, 56, 87, 94, 98, 111, 115

Gaia, 157
Gedulah (see Chesed), 51
Geburah, 33, 53, 54
Gemini, 33, 92, 117, 122
Gestalt therapy, 7
glove leather, 47
God, 3, 87, 125
goddesses, 79
god-forms, 117–122, 123
Godhead, xi, 8, 13, 37, 45, 79
god-names, 8
God-realization, 45
gods, 5, 32, 79
gold, xii, 119, 125, 137, 145
Golden Dawn, 69
Great Mother, 129
Great White Goddess, 5, 73
Greece, 94, 99
Greeks, xi, 65, 81, 83, 97, 99, 101, 107, 111, 116, 118, 125, 137
guided imagery, 7
guided visualization, 79

Hades, 97, 145, 156–157
Hatshepsut, Queen, 15
The Hanged Man, 33, 103
healing, 7, 130, 134, 146, 150, 152, 153
Hekate, 129
Henry VIII, 65
Hera, 16, 45, 111, 148, 149
Hermes, 4, 132–133
The Hermit, 33, 97–98
Herodotus, 16, 65
The Hierophant, 33, 91
hierosgamos, 149
Higher Self (see Self)
hippocrates, 81
Hod, 7, 33, 68–71, 83
Holy Guardian Angel, xii, 10
holy water, 34
Homer, 16, 65, 111
Huitzilpochtli, 125
hypnosis, 6, 7

I Ching, 80
imagination, xii, 1, 3, 4, 5, 6, 7, 10, 15, 20, 21, 32, 34, 63, 73, 79, 80, 117, 119, 129
immortality, 13
incense, 1, 5, 10, 15, 31, 34, 45, 46, 51, 59, 60, 63, 66, 69, 83, 94, 114, 115, 119, 120, 126, 145
India, 42, 59, 65, 66, 67, 74, 99, 106, 108, 111, 112

169

Isis, 45, 73, 129
Israel, 101

Japan, 85
Jews, 83, 99
Judgment, 114
Jung, C. G., 3, 7, 31, 122, 129
Jungian psychology, 12
Juno (Hera), 45, 148, 149
Jupiter, 33, 51, 100, 119, 120, 144–147

Kama, 74
karma, 101
Kether, 33, 36, 37, 38, 45
Krishna, 59, 89, 125
Kwan Yin, 129
kyphi, 46

Lady Sara (Cunningham-Carter), 125, 130, 133, 138, 142, 145, 149, 152, 155, 157
laurel, 87
leather, 47, 52, 53, 56–57, 105
Leo, 33, 96, 117, 119, 122
Levi, Eliphas, 117, 119
libido, 41
Libra, 33, 101, 117, 122
limbic system, 5
lion, xii
Logos, 41
Louis XIV, 70
The Lovers, 33, 92
love, 87, 92, 126, 130, 137, 138, 139, 146, 152
lust, 96

maceration, 13, 14
Madonna, 45, 129
magic, xi, 1, 3, 4, 7, 10, 15, 30, 32, 77, 117, 118
The Magician, 33, 133
Malkuth, 7, 33, 76, 77, 79, 80
Mars, 33, 55, 90, 104, 108, 119, 120, 140–142
massage oil, 25
matter, 12
Maya, 45
meditation, 8, 11, 12, 13, 37, 41, 59, 103, 126, 127, 130, 133, 134, 135, 138, 139, 142, 150, 153
Megalaion, 46
memory, 4, 5, 31
Mercury, 4, 33, 69, 83, 97, 109, 119, 120, 132, 133
Middle Pillar, 5, 6, 7, 8, 9
middle note, 26, 27, 126, 130, 134, 135, 138, 139, 142, 146, 150, 152
Mithras, 59, 125
Mohammed, 41, 65, 87
moon, 5, 31, 33, 73, 79, 86, 119, 120, 125, 130
The Moon, 33, 111, 128, 129
Moses, 81, 94, 114
Muses, 125
muscone, 42

musk deer, 41, 42
mynah bird, 112
myrtol, 87

Napoleon, 111
Neptune, 154–155
Nero, 65
Netzach, 7, 33, 55, 62, 63, 87, 108
NLP (Neurolinguistic programming, 4, 7

oil of Abramelin (see Abramelin)
olfaction, 2
onycha, 81, 94–95, 103
opium, 77
Oriental (base), 29, 91, 95, 100, 105, 106, 108, 126, 134, 135, 152
Osiris, 31, 59, 125
otto (see attar), 12, 16, 64, 65, 66, 109
Ovid, 101

Paracelsus, 3, 11
past-life regression, 138
pathworking, 79, 80
pentagram, 6
Persephone, 77, 97
Persia(ns), 73, 99, 106
phoenix, xii
Pisces, 33, 111, 117, 122
Pliny the Elder, 16, 59, 65, 81, 101
Pluto, 156–157
poleoresin, 26
poppy, 77, 122
Poseidon, 15, 145, 154–155
Potnia, 15
prana, 141
prefixation, 28
The Priestess, 33, 85
prima materia, 12
Pylos, 15
Pythagoras, 101

Qabala, xi, xii, 3, 5, 8, 10, 31, 32, 41, 45, 55, 59, 63, 69, 73, 77, 79, 81, 83, 85, 87, 89, 91, 92, 94, 96, 97, 99, 101, 103, 106, 107, 108, 109, 111, 112, 117, 125
Qabalistic Cross, 6
quintessence, 1, 3, 13

Ra, 46, 125
Ramses, 65
Regardie, Israel, 3, 6, 8, 10, 45
resin, 26
resin absolute, 23
resinoid, 22, 24
ritual, xi, 1, 4, 5, 6, 7, 8, 31
Romans, 87, 99, 101, 108
Rosicrucians, 65
Russian leather, 56

Sadi, 106
Sagittarius, 33, 106, 117, 122
Saladin, 65
Satir, Virginia, 4

Saturn, 33, 45, 79, 107, 109, 115, 119, 120, 121 148–150
Scorpio, 33, 104, 117, 119, 122
Selene, 129
Self, (higher), 1, 2, 3, 4, 5, 7, 8, 10, 11, 12, 13, 55, 59, 69, 80, 81, 99, 103, 107, 119
self-hypnosis, 6, 7
Self-realization, 1, 8, 59
sex, 112, 138
Shakespeare, 51
Shakti, 45
Sheba, Queen of, 46, 60
Shekinah, 45
silk, 34
Solomon, 3, 34, 46, 60, 99
solutio, 13
Solve et coagula, 11, 13
soul, 3, 6, 11, 12, 13, 31, 37, 45, 64, 67, 146, 155, 157
Spanish leather, 56, 57, 64, 67
Sphinx, 118–119
spirit, 12, 13, 31, 34, 41
The Star, 33, 109
Stellar Visions, 84, 88, 90, 91, 93, 96, 98, 102, 104, 111, 113, 115, 118
Stone, Philo, 145
Strength, 33, 96
styrene, 70
subconscious, xii, 1, 2, 4, 6, 20, 31, 73, 77, 78, 80, 121, 122, 157
sub rosa, 65
superconscious, 1, 2, 5, 108
Sun, 2, 31, 33, 96, 119, 120, 126
The Sun, 33, 112
Susinum, 46

tarot, 32, 80, 133
Taurus, 33, 91, 117, 119, 122
test strip, 21
Tetragrammaton, 34, 81
Third Eye, 41
Thoth, 4, 7, 133
thujone, 92
tiara, 74
Tibet, 41
tincture, 12, 38, 43, 45, 46, 47, 49, 60, 63, 70, 83, 99, 139
Tiphareth, xii, 7, 33, 59, 106, 114
top note, 26, 27, 88, 126, 130, 134, 135, 138, 139, 143, 150, 152
topaz, xii
The Tower, 33, 108
Tree of Life, xi, 3, 7, 8, 31, 32, 34, 37, 77, 79
Tuthankhamen, 15

unguent, 15, 89
United States, 87
Universal Mind, 37, 45
The Universe, 33, 115
Uranus, 151–153

Venus, 33, 63, 64, 87, 91, 101, 116, 119, 120, 136–137, 138

vermouth, 92
Virgil, 65, 111
Virgo, 33, 97, 117, 122
Vishnu, 65, 67, 89
visualization, 6, 8, 69, 79
voodoo, 78, 85, 102, 103, 109, 111, 115

water, 33, 117, 118, 119
whale, 37
Wheel of Fortune, 33, 99
White Goddess, (Great), 73, 79, 129
witchcraft, 42, 47, 49, 111, 121

Xenophon, 73

Yahweh, 149
Yang, 41, 125
Yesod, 7, 33, 72, 73, 79, 106
Yin, 125, 129
Yod, 98

Zeus, 16, 51, 60, 111 144, 145, 149
zibitone, 49
Zodiac 33, 117

BOOKS OF RELATED INTEREST

The Magical and Ritual Use of Herbs
by Richard Alan Miller

The Magical and Ritual Use of Aphrodisiacs
by Richard Alan Miller

The Healing Intelligence of Essential Oils
The Science of Advanced Aromatherapy
by Kurt Schnaubelt, Ph.D.

Advanced Aromatherapy
The Science of Essential Oil Therapy
by Kurt Schnaubelt, Ph.D.

The Encyclopedia of Aphrodisiacs
Psychoactive Substances for Use in Sexual Practices
by Christian Rätsch and Claudia Müller-Ebeling

Aromatherapy for Healing the Spirit
Restoring Emotional and Mental Balance with Essential Oils
by Gabriel Mojay

Hydrosols
The Next Aromatherapy
by Suzanne Catty

Secret Medicines from Your Garden
Plants for Healing, Spirituality, and Magic
by Ellen Evert Hopman

Inner Traditions • Bear & Company
P.O. Box 388
Rochester, VT 05767
1-800-246-8648
www.InnerTraditions.com

Or contact your local bookseller